VIROLOGY RESEARCH PROGRESS

ZIKA VIRUS SURVEILLANCE, VACCINOLOGY, AND ANTI-ZIKA DRUG DISCOVERY

COMPUTER-ASSISTED STRATEGIES TO COMBAT THE MENACE

VIROLOGY RESEARCH PROGRESS

Additional books and e-books in this series can be found on Nova's website under the Series tab.

VIROLOGY RESEARCH PROGRESS

ZIKA VIRUS SURVEILLANCE, VACCINOLOGY, AND ANTI-ZIKA DRUG DISCOVERY

COMPUTER-ASSISTED STRATEGIES TO COMBAT THE MENACE

SUBHASH C. BASAK
APURBA K. BHATTACHARJEE
AND
ASHESH NANDY
EDITORS

nova
Medicine & Health
New York

Library of Congress Cataloging-in-Publication Data

ISBN: 978-1-53614-970-8

Published by Nova Science Publishers, Inc. † New York

CONTENTS

PREFACE

"I shall be telling this with a sigh
Somewhere ages and ages hence:
Two roads diverged in a wood, and I—
I took the one less traveled by,
And that has made all the difference."
Robert Frost, The Road Not Taken

"Rational behavior requires theory. Reactive behavior requires only reflex action."
W. Edwards Deming

HIV/AIDS, Cholera, Bubonic plague, Smallpox, and Influenza (Flu) are some of the most brutal epidemics/ pandemics in human history killing hundreds of millions of people [1]. Pandemics and plagues also have considerable socioeconomic impact [2]. Parasitic diseases like malaria and leishmaniasis had taken millions of lives and continue to be virulent. The mosquito-borne human-infecting viruses, rotavirus and the seasonal influenza regularly affect lives across continents in the thousands and millions [3-5]. Of particular interest are the Flavivirus disease-inducing members - Yellow Fever Virus (YFV), West Nile Virus (WNV), Japanese Encephalitis Virus (JEV), Tick-borne Encephalitis Virus (TBEV), Dengue

Virus (DENV) and Zika Virus (ZIKV) [6]. The DENV falls within the category of neglected tropical diseases [7].

Zika Virus was first isolated from a febrile rhesus monkey in the Zika forest of Uganda in 1947 [3]. It drew our heightened attention following the large number of microcephaly in neonatal cases in the Latin Americas in 2015. On 1 February 2016, the World Health Organization (WHO) [3] declared that the recent association of Zika infection with clusters of microcephaly and other neurological disorders constituted a Public Health Emergency of International Concern. Although of late the severity and number of ZIKV afflicted cases have gone down, the public health community worldwide is keeping a watchful eye on it.

As compared to the earlier centuries, we have a larger repertoire of more diverse and fast acting technologies available at our hand today to manage and mitigate emerging diseases. Completion of the Human Genome Project has given rise to sequencing methods which can quickly determine the genetic sequence of a pathogen which produces alarming clinical pathologies. Following Moore's law, the power of computers, essential for data analysis and visualization, has grown substantially with time. The combination of genomic data of pathogens, modeling methods, and data driven methodologies can lead to a "***generic approach***" of surveillance, mitigation, and vaccine as well as drug design for emerging pathogens, the four pillars of which may consist of:

a) Epidemiological approaches for the characterization of reservoirs of next possible emerging pathogens,
b) Fast computational sequence comparison methods for the characterization of the emerging pathogens to understand how novel or severe they could be,
c) Once the sequences of the dominant strains have been determined, computer-aided vaccine design (CAVD) methods can be used to produce a set of probable vaccine candidates for quick synthesis/ production and testing in the laboratory,
d) Computer-assisted design of novel therapeutics and testing of new drugs or repurposing already existing FDA-approved drugs.

A battery of methods- *in vivo, in vitro* and *in silico*- will be needed to tackle viruses like the Zika virus [8-13]. As in many other fields of biomedical research, high throughput and low cost *in silico* technologies may provide the first line of defense against such emerging pathogens providing decision support systems for the judicious applications of medium throughput *in vitro* methods and low throughput as well as costly *in vivo* techniques.

An emerging trend in many scientific disciplines is a strong tendency of being transformed into some form of information science [14]. The editors of this book sincerely hope that the four-pronged computer-assisted approach mentioned above and described in more details in the chapters of this book will help in the management and mitigation of emerging infectious agents like the Zika.

REFERENCES

[1] Outbreak: 10 of the Worst Pandemics in History, *MPH Online*; https://www.mphonline.org/worst-pandemics-in-history/; Accessed on 12 November 2018.

[2] Bell, C. and Lewis, M. *The Economic Implications of Epidemics Old and New*; https://www.files.ethz.ch/isn/35778/2005_02_07.pdf; Accessed on 12 November 2018.

[3] *World Health Organization (WHO) report on Zika virus:* http://www.who.int/emergencies/zika-virus/mediacentre/press-releases/en/. (Accessed on 5 November 2018).

[4] Stenseth, N.C., Atshabar, B.B., Begon, M., Belmain, S.R., Bertherat, E., et al. 2008. "Plague: Past, present, and future." *PLoS Med* 5(1):3. doi:10.1371/journal.pmed.0050003

[5] Nandy, A. and Basak, S.C. 2016. "A Brief Review of Computer-Assisted Approaches to Rational Design of Peptide Vaccines." *Int. J. Mol. Sci.* 17(666). doi:10.3390/ijms17050666.

[6] Holbrook, M.R. 2017. "Historical Perspectives on Flavivirus Research." *Viruses* 9:97. doi:10.3390/v9050097.

[7] CDC *Report on neglected tropical diseases (NTD)*; https://www.cdc.gov/globalhealth/ntd/diseases/index.html; Accessed on 13 November 2018.

[8] Hamel, R., et al. 2015. "Biology of Zika Virus Infection in Human Skin Cells." *J Virol.* 89(17):8880–8896. doi: 10.1128/JVI.00354-15.

[9] Morrison, T.E. and Diamond, M.S. 2017. "Animal models of Zika virus infection, pathogenesis, and immunity." *J. Virol.* 91:e00009-17. https://doi.org/10.1128/JVI.00009-17.

[10] Marzi, A., Emanuel, J., Callison, J., McNally, K.L., et al. 2018. "Lethal Zika Virus Disease Models in Young and Older Interferon α/β Receptor Knock Out Mice." *Front. Cell. Infect. Microbiol.* 8:117. doi:10.3389/fcimb.2018.00117

[11] Papa, M.P., Meuren, L.M., Coelho, S.V.A., et al. 2017. "Zika Virus Infects, Activates, and Crosses Brain Microvascular Endothelial Cells, without Barrier Disruption." *Front. Microbiol.* 8:2557.doi:10.3389/fmicb.2017.02557

[12] Balasubramanian A, Teramoto T, Kulkarni AA, Bhattacharjee AK and Padmanabhan R (2017) Antiviral activities of selected antimalarials against dengue virus type and Zika virus. *Antiviral Research* 137:141-150.

[13] Bhattacharjee AK (2018) Pharmacophore modeling applied to mosquito-borne diseases. In: Devillers J (Ed), *Computational Design of Chemicals for the Control of Mosquitoes and Their Diseases*, CRC Press, Taylor & Francis Group, Boca Raton, FL, USA, pp. 139-169.

[14] *Statistical and Machine learning methods of network analysis*. 2012. Edited by M. Dehmer M. and Basak, S. C. New Jersey, USA: John Wiley & Sons.

In: Zika Virus Surveillance …
Editors: Subhash C. Basak et al.
ISBN: 978-1-53614-970-8

Chapter 1

ZIKA VIRUS: AN INTRODUCTION

Subhash C. Basak[1,*], PhD, Apurba Bhattacharjee[2], PhD, and Ashesh Nandy[3], PhD

[1]Department of Chemistry and Biochemistry, University of Minnesota Duluth, MN, US

[2]Biomedical Graduate Research Organization Department of Microbiology and Immunology School of Medicine, Georgetown University Washington, DC, US

[3]Centre for Interdisciplinary Research and Education, Kolkata, India

ABSTRACT

This first chapter by the three editors of the book provides an overview of the status of the Zika virus (ZIKV) with emphasis on: a) Discovery and brief history of Zika virus, b) Status of global Zika infection and transmission, c) Virology of the Zika virus, d) Clinical complications of the virus, e) Diagnosis of ZIKV, f) Biochemistry of ZIKV interaction with permissive cell types, and (g) Efforts in the discovery and design for anti-ZIKV drugs and vaccines. It specifically deals with a four-pronged approach, viz., data-driven epidemiological characterization of emerging pathogens, mathematical sequence descriptor based fast surveillance

---

* Corresponding Author E-mail: sbasak@d.umn.edu.

approaches, computer-assisted vaccine design, and computer-aided anti-Zika drug discovery to demonstrate how together the work can be an effective approach for the prevention, mitigation, and treatment of the Zika virus infection.

Keywords: Zika Virus (ZIKV), Viral Epidemics, Time to the most recent common ancestors (tMRCAs), The battle of Imphal, Antonine Plague or Plague of Galen, Untranslated Regions (UTRs), NS_5 RNA-dependent RNA polymerase, Exocytosis, Endocytosis, Phylogenetic tree, 2D graphical method, Guillain-Barré syndrome, Microcephaly, Reverse transcription-polymerase chain reaction (RT-PCR), Enzyme-linked immunosorbent assay (ELISA), Biomarker of Zika.

1. Discovery and Brief History

Viral epidemics often arise without warning and take humanity by surprise, sometimes with devastating consequences. The bubonic plague of Justinian (540-750 AD) killing 25-50% of the population of the known world, the Black Death plague of the fourteenth century that killed 20 to 30 million Europeans, the ravages of small pox in the Americas from the sixteenth century introduced by European soldiers and settlers that decimated many native populations, the Spanish Flu of 1918 that killed between 20-50 million people worldwide, the human immunodeficiency virus (HIV) that became a virulent pandemic leading to millions of incidences, among others, are noteworthy instances. The Zika virus (ZIKV) rampage in the Americas in 2015-17 is no exception [1].

The Zika virus came to occupy heightened attention following huge incidence of microcephaly in neo-natal cases in the Latin Americas in 2015. It was first isolated from a febrile rhesus monkey in the Zika forest (Figures 1.1 & 1.2) of Uganda in 1947 [2]. In 1952, the virus was isolated from humans. It then migrated through Africa and Asia and the first major outbreak of Zika infection was reported from the Island of Yap in the Federated States of Micronesia in 2007. The World Health Organization (WHO) report gives a brief history of the origin and spread of ZIKV.

Serosurvey of humans detected spreads of ZIKV throughout Africa, Asia, and Oceania. In 1954, the first three cases of ZIKV infection in humans were reported in Oyo state, Nigeria [3]. Fagbami [4] noted in his 1979 study that 40% of Nigerian adults and 25% of Nigerian children had antibodies of the virus.

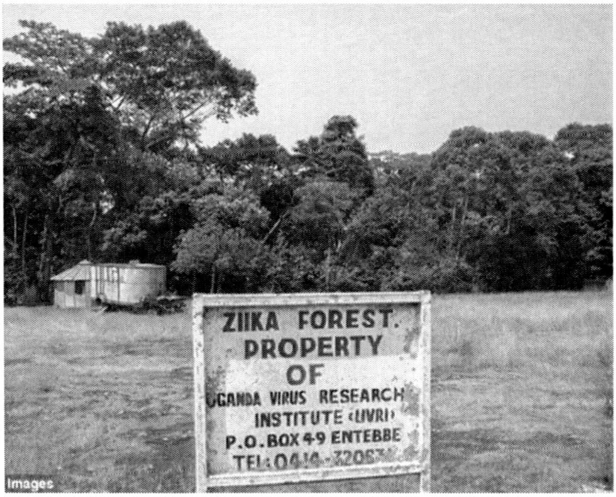
ZIIKA FOREST.
PROPERTY
OF
UGANDA VIRUS RESEARCH
INSTITUTE (UVRI)
P.O.BOX 49 ENTEBBE
Images

Figure 1.1. Zika Forest of Uganda.

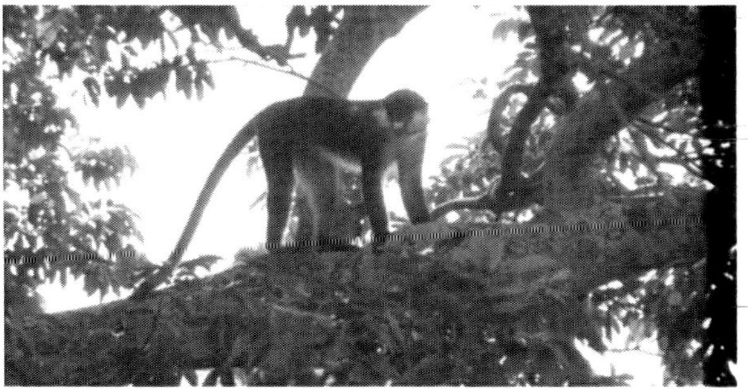

Figure 1.2. Picture of a rhesus monkey in the Zika Forest of Uganda. (Ref: https://images.search.yahoo.com/yhs/search?p=Zika+forest+of+Uganda+pictures&fr=yhs-adk-adk_sbnt&hspart=adk&hsimp=yhs-adk_sbnt&imgurl=http%3A%2F%2Fmarkacadeey.com%2Fwp-content%2Fuploads%2F2016%2F02%2FZIKA-FOREST-UGANDA.jpg#id=8&iurl=http%3A%2F%2Fi.dailymail.co.uk%2Fi%2Fpix%2F2016%2F02%2F02%2F13%2F30CF2AEA00000578-3428099-image-a-7_1454418507460.jpg&action=click).

Table 1. Zika virus detected from 1947, the pre-epidemic period [1]

Year	Country	Remarks
1947	Uganda	First isolation and identification of ZIKV. Found in rhesus monkey, R766, caged in Zika forest.
1948	Uganda	Detected in *A. africanus* mosquitoes. Found in Zika forest.
1951	Nigeria	First instance of ZIKV antibodies in human blood, found in children.
1952	Uganda, Tanganyika	First human cases of ZIKV infection detected.
	India	ZIKV antibodies found in human blood.
1953	Malaya, North Borneo, Philippines	ZIKV antibodies found in residents.
	Nigeria	ZIKV infection detected in three persons.
1954	Egypt, Vietnam	ZIKV antibodies found in few residents.
1955	Nigeria	ZIKV antibodies found in human blood.
1957	Mozambique	ZIKV antibodies found in human blood.
1958	Uganda	Two strains of ZIKV found in *A. aegypti* mosquitoes in Zika forest.
1960	Angola	ZIKV antibodies found in indigenous residents.
1961-62	Central African Republic	ZIKV antibodies found in human blood.
1961-64	Ethiopia	ZIKV antibodies found in human blood.
1962	Senegal	ZIKV antibodies found in human blood.
1963-64	Central African Republic, Burkina-Faso	ZIKV antibodies found in human blood.
1963-65	Ivory Coast	ZIKV antibodies found in human blood.
1964	Uganda	First confirmation that ZIKV causes human disease. Clinical features reported.
1964-65	Guinea-Bissau	ZIKV antibodies found in human blood.
1964-66	Togo, Cameroon	ZIKV antibodies found in human blood.
1965	Niger	ZIKV antibodies found in human blood.

Year	Country	Remarks
1965-67	Nigeria	ZIKV antibodies found in human blood.
1967	Benin, Gabon, Liberia	ZIKV antibodies found in human blood.
1966-67	Uganda, Kenya, Somalia, Morocco	ZIKV antibodies found in human blood.
1967-69	Uganda	ZIKV antibodies found in human blood.
1968	Kenya	ZIKV antibodies found in human blood.
1969-72	Nigeria	ZIKV antibodies found in human blood.
1969	Malaysia	ZIKV found in *A. aegypti* mosquitoes.
1969-83	Indonesia, Malaysia, Pakistan	ZIKV found in mosquitoes. Sporadic human infections.
1970	Nigeria	ZIKV antibodies found in human blood.
1971-72	Angola	ZIKV antibodies found in human blood.
1972, 1975, 1988, 1990	Senegal	ZIKV antibodies found in human blood.
1979	Central African Republic	ZIKV antibodies found in human blood.
1980	Nigeria	ZIKV antibodies found in human blood.
1984	Uganda	ZIKV antibodies found in human blood.
1996-97	Malaysia	ZIKV antibodies found in human blood.
1999	Ivory Coast	ZIKV antibodies found in human blood.

A. africanus, Aedes africanus; ZIKV, Zika virus.

Table 2. ZIKV epidemics, 2007 to present

Year	Country	Remarks
2007	Yap Island, Micronesia	First outbreak reported in humans.
2008	Senegal	First reported case of traveler infected in Senegal returning to home country and passing infection through sexual contact.
2010	Cameroon	ZIKV antibodies found in human blood.

Table 2. (Continued)

Year	Country	Remarks
2010-2015	Cambodia, Indonesia, Malaysia, Philippines, Thailand, Maldives	Mosquito transmission of ZIKV in these countries to travelers who then carried the infection to their home countries.
2011-2014	French Polynesia	Second reported outbreak of ZIKV infections. Connection with microcephaly and neurological disorders established later.
2013-2014	Chile, Cook Islands, New Caledonia	ZIKV outbreak.
2013	Tahiti	ZIKV isolated from patient's semen showing sexual transmissibility.
2014	Zambia	ZIKV antibodies found in human blood.
2015 April/May	Brazil, Bahia state	National Reference Laboratory, Brazil confirmed, by PCR, ZIKV infections, for the first time in the Americas
2015 July	Brazil	Zika cases confirmed by laboratory tests in 12 states. Neurological disorders associated with prior viral infections detected primarily in the Bahia region.
2015 October	South America	Colombia, Republic of Cabo Verde report confirmed cases of ZIKV infections. Brazil reported unusual increase in the number of cases of neonatal microcephaly.
2015 November	Central and South America	Brazil reported 141 suspected cases of microcephaly and declared a national public health emergency. Brazil reported detection of ZIKV in amniotic fluid of fetuses with confirmed microcephaly.

Year	Country	Remarks
		Suriname, Panama, El Salvador, Guatemala and Paraguay confirmed cases of ZIKV infection. The Pan American Health Organization and WHO issued an epidemiological alert.
2015 November	Mexico	Three cases of ZIKV infection confirmed by PCR.
2015 November	French Polynesia	Retrospective analysis reveals unusually large number of central nervous system malformations in fetuses and infants in 2014-2015.
2015 December	Central and South America	Honduras, French Guiana and Martinique reported confirmed cases of ZIKV infections.
2015 December	Puerto Rico	First confirmed case of Zika infection reported.
2016	Maldives	Finnish national working in Maldives tested positive for Zika after return to Finland.
2016 January	Americas	Guyana reported the first PCR-confirmed case of locally acquired Zika infection. Ecuador, Bolivia, Barbados, Haiti, Dominican Republic, Nicaragua, Curacao and Jamaica reported the first confirmed cases of Zika infections. First case of Zika in St. Martin reported.
2016 January	US Virgin Islands	First confirmed case of Zika in St. Croix reported.
2016 February	Americas	First confirmed case of ZIKV infection in Chile reported. First case of sexually transmitted Zika infection in Texas, USA reported.

Table 2. (Continued)

Year	Country	Remarks
2016	Various countries	Angola, Antigua, British Virgin Islands, Trinidad and Tobago, Guadeloupe, Fiji, Marshall Islands, Papua New Guinea, and other countries report first cases of ZIKV infections.
2016	Singapore	ZIKV infection reported.
2016/2017	India	Three cases of ZIKV infection reported in Ahmedabad.
2017	Singapore	Several cases of locally transmitted ZIKV confirmed.

Data summarized from source: (1): Kindhauser, M. K., Allen T., Frank, V., Santhana, R. S. and Dye, C. Zika: the origin and spread of a mosquito-borne virus. Bull World Health Organ.

2016;94(9):675–686C. doi:10.2471/BLT.16.171082; 2) WHO Situation Report on Zika Virus, 9th March 2017 http://apps.who.int/iris/bitstream/10665/254714/1/zikasitrep10Mar17-eng.pdf?ua=1.

Tables 1 and 2 provide data on: a) the cases of ZIKV detected during the pre-epidemic period (1947 to 1999) and b) the case history of ZIKV during 2007 to 2017, respectively.

As the epidemic progressed the number of cases in the regions of the Western hemisphere increased. Table 3 below summarizes the number of cases of ZIKV infection in the regions of the Americas detected up to 11 May 2017.

On 2 March 2015 Brazil notified WHO of reports of an illness characterized by skin rash in northeastern states. From February 2015 to 29 April 2015, nearly 7000 cases of illness with skin rash were reported in these states. All cases were mild, with no reported deaths. Zika was not suspected at that stage, and no tests for Zika were carried out. On 1 February 2016, WHO [2] declared that the recent association of Zika infection with clusters of microcephaly and other neurological disorders constituted a Public Health Emergency of International Concern. It should be mentioned that WHO later relaxed this warning subsequently in November of the same year.

Table 3. Cumulative cases of ZIKV infection in the Americas 2015-2017 as of 11 May 2017

Region*	Confirmed autochthonus cases	Imported cases	Deaths from ZIKV infection	Confirmed congenital syndrome associated with ZIKV infection
North America	225	5478	0	67
Latin America (Mexico)	8731	15	0	5
Central American Isthmus	6309	77	0	81
Latin Caribbean	41823	205	5	143
Andean area	15136	41	0	167
Brazil	133527	0	11	2653
Southern cone	100	75	0	4
Non-Latin Caribbean	5649	29	4	10
TOTAL	211500	5920	20	3130

*Regions defined as follows: North America: Bermuda, Canada, United States of America; Central American Isthmus: Belize, Costa Rica, El Salvador, Guatemala, Honduras, Nicaragua, Panama; Latin Caribbean: Cuba, Dominican Republic, French Guiana, Guadeloupe, Haiti, Martinique, Puerto Rico, St Barthelemy, St Martin; Andean Region: Bolivia, Colombia, Ecuador, Peru; Southern cone: Argentina, Chile, Paraguay, Uruguay; Non-Latin Caribbean: Anguilla, Antigua and Barbuda, Aruba, Bahamas, Barbados, Bonaire, St Eustatius and Saba, Cayman Islands, Curacao, Dominica, Grenada, Guyana, Jamaica, Montserrat, St Kitts and Nevis, St Lucia, St Vincent and the Grenadines, St Maarten, Suriname, Trinidad and Tobago, Turks and Caicos Islands, Virgin Islands (UK), Virgin Islands (USA).

Data summarized from source: Pan American Health Organization/World Health Organization. Zika suspected and confirmed cases reported by countries and territories in the Americas Cumulative cases, 2015–2017. Updated as of 11 May 2017. Washington, D.C.: PAHO/WHO; 2017; Pan American Health Organization • www.paho.org • © PAHO/WHO, 2017.

Liang et al. [5] carried out computational analysis of ZIKV evolution, nucleotide substitution rate and the time to the most recent common ancestors (tMRCAs). These authors proposed that a "global dissemination of ZIKV spread was likely to have originated from Africa, followed by eastward transmission to South-eastern Asia, Oceania, South America, Caribbean and Central America." Regarding the spread of the virus from Africa to Asia, the authors had the following interesting observations:

> "Relatively few studies on the origin of the South Pacific Rim lineage had been reported in the literature. The tMRCA for South Pacific Rim was estimated to be 1947 (95% HPD interval.35 to 1966) in our study. Coincidentally, during the Second World War in South-eastern Asia, around 100,000 East and West African soldiers were brought into combat in the Burma Campaign from January 1942 to July 1945. Specifically, the British Empire colonial unit 11th (East Africa) Infantry Division comprised troops from East and West African countries such as Kenya, Uganda, Nyasaland, Tanganyika and Rhodesia (Burma Star Association-- The 11th East African Division). During those three-years' conflict, both sides suffered heavy casualties, including at least 20,000 Japanese soldiers who died because of disease in the *battle of Imphal*. It is also noteworthy that Thai army was also involved in this campaign and that after the Japanese surrendered, troops were continued to be deployed to the then Malaya. The whole campaign could serve as a possible portal of entry for the transmission of ZIKV from Africa to South-eastern Asia during that wartime period."

This scenario of infectious disease transmission is not without precedents. The first incidences of possibly smallpox in Europe was the Antonine Plague of 165 to 180 AD, also known as the Plague of Galen (from the name of the Greek physician living in the Roman Empire who described it), was an ancient pandemic brought back to the Roman Empire by troops returning from the Near East campaigns [6]. The Plague of Justinian (541–542 AD) afflicted the Eastern Roman (Byzantine) Empire, especially its capital Constantinople, the Sasanian Empire, and port cities around the entire Mediterranean. It probably originated in Ethiopia and came through rodents in ships carrying grain to Rome. Smallpox infections that decimated the native populations of the New World was carried there by the Spanish conquistadores [7]; in turn syphilis was carried eastwards from the New World to Europe and thence the whole world. Currently, pandemic viruses gain increasingly rapid circulation through globalization and worldwide fast travels in our inter-connected world.

2. Status of Global Zika Infection and Transmission

Viral epidemics and pandemics at the initial stage grow very fast, then after a period of a few months fall into quiescence as the populations get herd immunity or the virus itself mutates away from its destructive form. Often as in the case of the bubonic plague, or the H1N1 influenza, the virus may start another round of epidemic and the process goes on and on.

Following a similar trend, of late, the Zika epidemic has lost its severity. Governments that had issued travel advisories at the height of the ZIKV pandemic have revised the advisories, but still caution against travel to Zika infested areas. Here is the current CDC Zika Travel Advisory and Information [8].

2.1. Areas with Risk of Zika

Because Zika infection during pregnancy can cause severe birth defects, pregnant women should not travel to the areas below. Partners of pregnant women and couples considering pregnancy should know the risks to pregnancy and take prevention steps. All travelers should strictly follow steps to prevent mosquito bites and prevent sexual transmission during and after the trip.

Africa

Angola, Benin, Burkina-Faso, Burundi, Cameroon, Cape Verde, Central African Republic, Chad, Congo (Congo-Brazzaville), Côte d'Ivoire, Democratic Republic of the Congo (Congo-Kinshasa), Equatorial Guinea, Gabon, Gambia, Ghana, Guinea, Guinea-Bissau, Kenya, Liberia, Mali, Niger, Nigeria, Rwanda, Senegal, Sierra Leone, South Sudan, Sudan, Tanzania, Togo, Uganda.

Asia

Bangladesh, Burma (Myanmar), Cambodia, India, Indonesia, Laos, Malaysia, Maldives, Pakistan, Philippines, Singapore, Thailand, Timor-Leste (East Timor), Vietnam

The Caribbean

Anguilla; Antigua and Barbuda; Aruba; Barbados; Bonaire; British Virgin Islands; Cuba; Curaçao; Dominica; Dominican Republic; Grenada; Haiti; Jamaica; Montserrat; the Commonwealth of Puerto Rico, a US territory; Saba; Saint Kitts and Nevis; Saint Lucia; Saint Martin; Saint Vincent and the Grenadines; Saint Eustatius; Saint Maarten; Trinidad and Tobago; Turks and Caicos Islands; US Virgin Islands

Central America

Belize, Costa Rica, El Salvador, Guatemala, Honduras, Nicaragua, Panama

North America

Mexico

The Pacific Islands

Fiji, Papua New Guinea, Samoa, Solomon Islands, Tonga

South America

Argentina, Bolivia, Brazil, Colombia, Ecuador, French Guiana, Guyana, Paraguay, Peru, Suriname, Venezuela

2.2. Areas with Interrupted Transmission

Zika was previously found in the locations on this list, but scientists have determined the virus is no longer present. This means all travelers, including pregnant women, can visit these destinations with no known risk of getting Zika from mosquitoes. If Zika returns to a country or territory on this list, CDC will remove it from the list and post updated information. Check this page for the most up-to-date information before making travel plans.

We give below the information regarding the geographical area and the date of Interruption [8].

Area	Date of interruption
American Samoa	13 April 2017
The Bahamas	2 February 2018
Cayman Islands	20 July 2017
Cook Islands	10 March 2017
Guadeloupe	29 June 2017
French Polynesia	10 March 2017
Isla de Pascua, Chile	10 March 2017
Marshall Islands	9 January 2018
Martinique	29 June 2017
Micronesia	23 November 2017
New Caledonia	10 March 2017
Palau	23 November 2017
Saint Barthélemy	24 May 2017
Vanuatu	10 March 2017

3. Virology of the Zika Virus

The Zika virus belongs to the Flavivirus genus that is part of the family Flaviviridae. Some important disease-causing viruses of this genus are Dengue fever virus, Tick-borne encephalitis virus, West Nile virus, Japanese encephalitis virus, and Zika virus [9]. The viruses of this group contain a single stranded positive sense RNA genome containing about 11,000 nucleotides [10]. Consequently, the RNAs of such viruses can be directly translated to a large polyprotein that is subsequently converted by viral and host cell proteases into two sets of proteins: Structural and nonstructural. The three structural proteins are: Envelope, E; membrane precursor, PrM; and capsid, C (Figure 1.3). These are critical for the formation of the capsid and envelop of the mature virus. The seven non-structural (NS) proteins, on the other hand, have important roles in the replication of the virus. The NS group of proteins include: NS1, NS2a, NS2b, NS3, NS4a, NS4b, and NS5 as shown in Figure 1.3 [11].

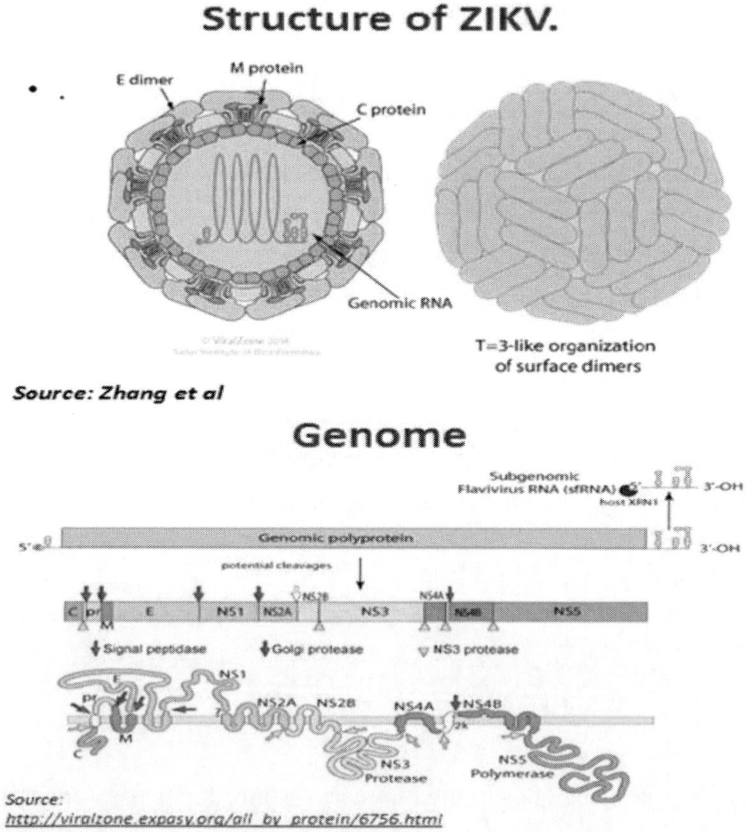

Figure 1.3. The three structural proteins and seven non-structural (NS) proteins of Flaviviruses.

Table 4. Structure of a typical flavivirus genome including UTRs

Srl No	Gene	Sequence span,nt	Sequence length*	Protein/Biological function
1	5'-UTR	1-107	107	Encodes regions essential for genome cyclization/replication.
2	Capsid	108-473	366	Virion structure.
3	prM/M	474-977	504	prM forms heterodimers with E to form immature virion. prM then cleaved and mature virions formed with M.
4	E	978-2489	1512	Viral entry into host cell.
5	NS1	2490-3545	1056	Viral replication, immune evasion, genome synthesis.
6	NS2A	3546-4223	678	Transmembrane protein, part of replication complex; assembly/secretion of virus particles.
7	NS2B	4224-4613	390	Cofactor for proteinase domain of NS3; proteolytic processing.
8	NS3	4614-6464	1851	Protease/helicase.
9	NS4A	6465-6914	381	Viral RNA replication and amplification.
10	2K	6846-6914	69	Peptide generated by cleavage at the N terminus of the NS4B signal sequence.
11	NS4B	6915-7667	753	Facilitates viral replication complexes; counteracts innate immune responses.
12	NS5	7668-10376	2709	Methyltransferase; RNA-dependent RNA polymerase.
13	3'-UTR	10380-10807	427	Facilitates viral replication and translation.

* Typical length data taken from ZIKV isolate ZIKV/*H.sapiens*/Brazil/PE243/2015 (GenBank Locus ID KX197192), complete genome. E, envelope; NS, non-structural; nt, nucleotide; prM/M, pre-membrane/membrane; UTR, untranslated region.

Table 4 summarizes the structure of Flavivirus genome including the untranslated regions, 5’-UTR and 3’-UTR regions [1, 11].

The 3’ terminus has a sub-genomic Flavivirus RNA (sfRNA) structure that is essential for causing disease in humans [12, 13]. The envelope protein comprises most of the virion surface and participates in viral-host cell binding and membrane fusion during replication.

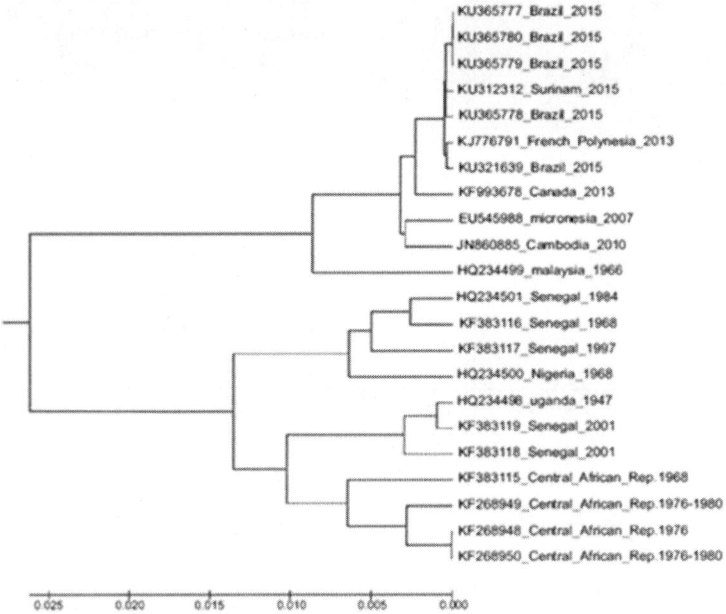

Figure 1.4. Phylogenetic tree of 22 ZIKV genome sequences. Nandy et al.16. Reproduced with permission from Bentham Science Publishers, www.benthamscience.com.ZIKV, Zika virus.

Replication of ZIKV, like other Flaviviruses, occurs in the cytoplasm of infected cells [14, 15]. After endocytosis mediated by a still unknown cellular receptor, viral fusion occurs with endosomal membranes. This results in the uncoating of the viral particle and release of the viral genome. The genome is subsequently translated into a single polyprotein at the endoplasmic reticulum (ER). The polyprotein is processed by viral NS2B–NS3 protease and other cellular proteases generating mature viral proteins. The positive-sense viral RNA genome is then copied to produce a negative-sense RNA molecule chain, which is used as the template for synthesis of the full length positive-sense viral genomic RNA. Synthesis of viral genome occurs in association with the ER and is catalyzed by a replication complex consisting of NS5 RNA-dependent RNA polymerase and other NS proteins. The new genomes are packaged by the C protein; they acquire envelopes while budding from the ER. These immature virions thus produced are translocated through the cellular secretory pathways, where E glycosylation and cleavage of prM by host furin protease occurs producing the mature virions that are released by exocytosis.

From its initial stage in Uganda, the ZIKV has undergone quite a few changes. Figure 1.4 gives a phylogenetic tree of 22 ZIKV sequences [16].

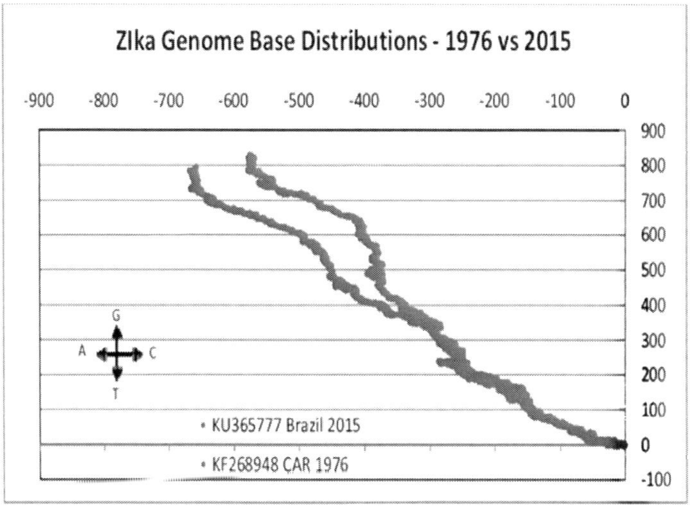

Figure 1.5. Comparison of ZIKV genomes from Central African Republic 1976 to Brazil 2015 in 2D graphical representation16. Axes AGCT as shown in the inset. The algorithm involved starting at the origin and plotting a point for each base in the nucleotide sequence by a step in the xy-plane defined by A(-1,0), C(+1,0), G(0,+1), T(0,-1) until the end of the sequence, thus plotting a graph that reflects the base distribution and composition of the sequence. Figure reproduced with permission from Bentham Science Publishers, www.benthamscience.com.2D, two-dimensional; ZIKV, Zika virus.

Although the typical nucleotide sequences provide a complete description of the linear arrangement of the bases in the gene, graphical representation methods [17] may lead to visualization of the differences among sequences. Figure 1.5 shows such a representation of ZIKV genomes from Central African Republic 1976 to Brazil 2015 by the 2D graphical method developed by one of the authors of this chapter (Nandy) for compact representation and visualization of nucleic acidsequences [17].

4. Clinical Complications and Zika Virus

4.1. Clinical Signs and Symptoms

The Centers for Disease Control and Prevention [18] gives s detailed list of information about the clinical aspects of the Zika virus infection.

Many people infected with Zika virus do not develop many overt systems. The symptoms where they do develop last for several days to a week. However, there have been cases of Guillain-Barré syndrome reported in patients after Zika virus infection. It has been concluded by CDC that Zika virus infection during pregnancy is associated with microcephaly and other severe fetal brain defects. Due to this concern for microcephaly arising out of maternal Zika virus infection, fetuses and infants of women infected with Zika virus during pregnancy should be evaluated for possible congenital infection and neurologic abnormalities.

4.2. Zika and Guillain-Barre Syndrome

Another complication of ZIKV infection is its association with the Guillain-Barré syndrome (GBS), a neurological disorder [19-21].

The exact cause of Guillain-Barré syndrome is unknown. It can occur a few days or weeks after the person has had symptoms of a respiratory or gastrointestinal viral infection. Occasionally, surgery will trigger the syndrome. In rare instances, vaccinations may increase the risk of GBS. Recently, some countries around the world have reported an increased incidence of GBS following infection with the Zika virus.

As is well known, currently there is no available cure for GBS [22]. Some therapeutic interventions can only decrease the severity of disease and shorten recovery time.

4.3. Risk Factors for Zika Virus [18]

Factors that put a person at greater risk of developing Zika virus disease include:

Living in or traveling to areas where there have been ZIKV outbreaks. Being in tropical and subtropical areas increases the risk of exposure to the Zika virus disease.

Having unprotected sex. Isolated cases of sexually transmitted Zika virus have been reported. The CDC advises abstinence from sexual activity during pregnancy or condom use during all sexual contact for men with a pregnant sex partner if the man has traveled to an area of active Zika virus transmission.

5. Modes of Transmission of Zika Virus

Current CDC website gives the following information regarding the transmission of the ZIKV transmission [23].

Zika virus can spread in various ways described below [23, 24]:

Through mosquito bites: Zika virus is transmitted to people primarily through the bite of infected mosquitoes (Ae. aegypti or Ae. albopictus). Mosquitoes become infected when they feed on a person already infected with the virus. Infected mosquitoes can then spread the virus to other people through bites.

From mother to child: A pregnant woman can pass Zika virus to her fetus during pregnancy.

Through sex: Zika can be passed through sex from a person who has Zika to his or her partners. Zika can be passed through sex, even if the infected person does not have symptoms at the time. It can be passed from a person with Zika before their symptoms start, while they have symptoms, and after their symptoms end.

Through blood transfusion: There have been multiple reports of blood transfusion transmission cases in Brazil. These reports are currently being investigated.

During the French Polynesian outbreak, 2.8% of blood donors tested positive for Zika and in previous outbreaks, the virus has been found in blood donors.

Through laboratory and healthcare setting exposure:

Prior to the current outbreak, there were four reports of laboratory acquired Zika virus infections, although the route of transmission was not clearly established in all cases.

As of June 15, 2016, there has been one reported case of laboratory-acquired Zika virus disease in the United States [23].

To date, no cases of confirmed Zika virus transmission in healthcare settings have been reported in the United States. Recommendations are available for healthcare providers to help prevent exposure to Zika virus in healthcare settings.

6. Diagnosis of Zika Virus

The diagnosis and isolation of ZIKV is a complex process which includes assays such as reverse transcription-polymerase chain reaction (RT-PCR), real-time qRT-PCR, loop-mediated isothermal amplification (LAMP), lateral flow assays (LFAs), biosensors, nucleic acid sequence-based amplification (NASBA) tests, strand invasion-based amplification tests, and immune assays like enzyme-linked immunosorbent assay (ELISA). The readers are advised to consult the relevant literature on the subject [25, 26].

7. ZIKV Interaction with Permissive Cell Types

ZIKV is a versatile infective agents and attacks different types of permissive cells in the human body using multiple mechanisms. In Table 5 we give a few examples of how ZIKV interacts with various permissive cell types.

Table 5. Examples of ZIKV infection and entry into different types of cells

Cell/Tissue	Virus source/strain	Mechanism of entry	Literature source
Human dermal fibroblasts, epidermal keratinocytes and immature dendritic cells	ZIKV isolate, from French Polynesia	Entry and/or adhesion factors included DC-SIGN1, AXL, Tyro3, and, to a lesser extent, TIM-1, permitted ZIKV entry, with a major role for the TAM receptor AXL.	Ref [27]
Human microglia and astrocytes	$ZIKV^{BR}$	Activates AXL kinase activity, which downmodulates interferon signaling	Ref [28]
Vero cells, human brain microvascular endothelial cells, human neural stem cells, and mouse neutrospheres.	ZIKV strain MR 766 (Uganda/Africa, accession no.: NC012532.1	Entry of ZIKV inhibited by Chloroquine	Ref [29]

As is clear from data [27-29] in Table 5 above and other studies [30-32], ZIKV uses a diverse set of biochemical mechanisms to infect the target cells.

CONCLUSION

From its initial reservoir in the Zika forest of Uganda ZIKV has spread into large parts of the globe which includes Asia, other parts of Africa, the Caribbean, Central America, The Pacific Islands, and South America. Currently, the virus has two dominant subtypes: a) Southern-Eastern Asian type and b) African type. It can attack different organs of the human body and cause multiple short-term and long-term pathologies. ZIKV enters human cells and interacts with them using a multiplicity of mechanisms. Understanding the mechanisms of ZIKV- human cell interactions at the ultrastructural and biochemical levels may lead not only to more thorough understanding of Zika virus virology, but also to intervention strategies through rational vaccine design as well as novel drug discovery.

One interesting area of research in ZIKV biochemistry is the discovery of biomarkers [33] associated with infection by the virus and subsequent pathological conditions. This may help in an in-depth understanding of ZIKV mediated pathological processes.

In view of the frequent occurrence of emerging pathogens in recent times, we need to focus research on the characterization of reservoirs of next possible pathogens. This aspect tis covered in chapter 5 of this book. Once the emerging outbreak of virus has been identified, it must be sequenced quickly to understand what type it is and by which molecular mechanisms it spreads through human populations and how it affects the infected individuals. Fast computational sequence comparison methods are needed for this purpose and this aspect is discussed in chapter 4 of the book.

Currently, no drug or vaccine is known for treatment of ZIKV. For emerging pathogens like the ZIKV, we need both vaccine and new drugs that can prevent the infection and treat the clinical symptoms produced by the virus. Chapter 2 and 3 cover these two aspects. Chapter 2 covers computer-assisted discovery and design of potential anti-ZIKV drugs and Chapter 3 discusses computer-assisted design of peptide vaccines for prevention against Zika virus.

Discovery of a new drug takes about 10 to 15 years and costs over two billion US dollars [34, 35]. Therefore, any technology that can improve the efficiency of the process is highly valuable to this endeavor. Computer aided drug discovery thus plays a pivotal role in bringing new potential anti-ZIKV drug to the forefront for this effort. Since no antiviral drug is currently available for tackling ZIKV, a fast track approach is necessary to counter the menacing movement of the virus. One quick approach could be "*repurposing*" of existing or abandoned drugs and shortlisting them using computational methods to circumvent the urgent need for anti-ZIKV drugs. Novel uses of already existing drugs will cost much less as compared to the pursuit of new drug discovery process. A successful recent attempt was reported through anti-ZIKV testing of 774 Food and Drug Administration (FDA) approved drugs [36]. The knowledge contained in these compounds can further be utilized in combination with chemoinformatic tools to develop models for harnessing the advantage toward more effective discovery of anti-ZIKV drugs. Pharmacophore based screening is one such tool that can be effective since the target structure of proteins involved in ZIKV virus is still uncertain. Since pharmacophore transcends the chemical structural class and captures only the features responsible for activity, use of pharmacophore has the advantage for identification of potentially new biologically active compounds of novel chemical scaffolds to open new chapters for chemotherapy of ZIKV [37, 38].

This book describes a holistic approach to the Zika virus problem involving characterization of reservoirs, surveillance of pathogens using genomics well as sequence comparison methodologies, vaccine design for the prevention of infection, and computer-assisted drug discovery.

REFERENCES

[1] Nandy, A. and Basak, S. C. (2017) The Epidemic that Shook the World—The Zika Virus Rampage, *Exploratory Research and Hypothesis in Medicine.* 2: 43–56.

[2] *World Health Organization (WHO) report on Zika virus:* http://www.who.int/emergencies/zika-virus/mediacentre/press-relea

ses/en/;http://www.who.int/emergencies/zika-virus/timeline/en/ (Accessed on 28 October 2018).

[3] MacNamara F. N. (1954) Zika virus: a report on three cases of human infection during an epidemic of jaundice in Nigeria. *Trans R Soc Trop Med Hyg*. 48:1 -145.

[4] Fagbami A. H. (1979) Zika virus infection in Nigeria: virology and seroepidemological investigation in Oyo stae. *Journal of Hygiene*. 83: 213-219.

[5] Liang D., Leung, R. K. K., Lee, S. S. and Kam KM (2017) Insights into intercontinental spread of Zika virus. *PLoS ONE* 12(4): e0176710. https://doi.org/10.1371/journal.pone.0176710.

[6] Verity Murphy, V. (2005). *Past pandemics that ravaged Europe;* http://news.bbc.co.uk/2/hi/health/4381924.stm; Accessed on 28 October 2018.

[7] Pringle, H. (2015). *How Europeans brought sickness to the New World*; June 4, 2015; https://www.sciencemag.org/news/2015/06/how-europeans-brought-sickness-new-world; Accessed on 28 October 2018.

[8] *Centers for Disease Control and Prevention*, https://wwwnc.cdc.gov/travel/page/zika-travel-information (Accessed on 29 October 2018).

[9] Armstrong, N., Hou, W. and Tang, Q. (2017) Biological and historical overview of Zika virus, *World J Virol*. 6(1): 1–8.

[10] Faye, O., Freire, C. C., Iamarino, A., Faye, O., de Oliveira, J. V., Diallo, M., Zanotto, P. M. and, Sall A. A. (2014) Molecular evolution of Zika virus during its emergence in the 20(th) century. *PLoS Negl Trop Dis* 8: e2636 [PMID: 24421913 DOI: 10.1371/journal.pntd.0002636].

[11] Ng, W. C., Soto-Acosta, R., Bradrick, S. S Mariano A., Garcia-Blanco, M. A. and Ooi, E. E. (2017) The 50 and 30 Untranslated Regions of the Flaviviral Genome, *Viruses* 9, 137; doi:10.3390/v9060137.

[12] Okafor, I. I., Ezugwu, F. O. and, Ekwochi, U. (2016) *Zika Virus: The Emerging Global Health Challenge, Diversity and Equality in Health and Care,* 13(6): 394-401.

[13] Clarke, B. D., Roby, J. A., Slonchak, A. and Khromykh, A. A. (2015) Functional non-coding RNAs derived from the flavivirus 3′ untranslated region. *Virus Res*. 206: 53-61.

[14] Barzon, L., Trevisan, M., Sinigaglia, A., Lavezzo, E. and Palù G. (2016) Zika virus: from pathogenesis to disease control. *FEMS Microbiol Lett*. Sep;363(18). pii: fnw202. Epub 2016 Aug 21.

[15] Suthar, M. S., Diamond, M. S. and Gale, M., Jr. (2013) West Nile virus infection and immunity. *Nat Rev Microbiol*., 11:115–28.

[16] Nandy, A., Dey, S., Basak, S. C., Bielinska-Waz, D. and Waz P. (2016) Characterizing the Zika Virus Genome – A Bioinformatics Study. *Curr. Comp.-Aided Drug Des.,* 12: 87-97.

[17] Nandy, A. (1994) A new graphical representation and analysis of DNA sequence structure: I. Methodology and Application to Globin Genes. *Current Si.,* 66(4): 309-314.

[18] Centers for Disease Control and Prevention. *CDC.* https://www.cdc.gov/zika/hc-providers/preparing-for-zika/clinicalevaluation disease. html; Accessed on 29 October 2018.

[19] Cao-Lormeau, V. M. et al. (2016) Guillain-Barré Syndrome outbreak associated with Zika virus infection in French Polynesia: a case-control study. *Lancet,* 9;387(10027):1531-1539. doi: 10.1016/S0140-6736(16)00562-6. Epub 2016 Mar 2.

[20] Beatriz Parra, B. et al. (2016) Guillain–Barré Syndrome Associated with Zika Virus Infection in Colombia. *N Engl J Med*, 375:1513-1523 DOI: 10.1056/NEJMoa1605564.

[21] WHO report on: Zika Virus, Microcephaly and 28) Guillain–Barré Syndrome. *WHO.* http://apps.who.int/iris/bitstream/handle/10665/204609/zikasitrep_10Mar2016_eng.pdf;jsessionid=F9E4895E617656 2081D34C0DED1A6550?sequence=1.

[22] NIH Guillain-Barré Syndrome Fact Sheet. *NIH.* https://www.ninds.nih.gov/Disorders/Patient-Caregiver-Education/Fact-Sheets/Guillain-Barr%C3%A9-Syndrome-Fact-Sheet; Accessed on 29 October 2018.

[23] Zika virus transmission methods, *CDC*. https://www.cdc.gov/zika/prevention/transmission-methods.html (Accessed on29 October 2018).

[24] Kaur, M., Gupte, S. and Kaur, T. (2016) Emergence of Zika Virus Infection. *J Hum Virol Retrovirol* 3(5): 00108. DOI: 10.15406/jhvrv.2016.03.00108.

[25] Singh, R. K., Dhama, K., Karthik, K., Tiwari, R., Khandia, R., Munjal, A., Iqbal H. M. N., Malik, Y. S. and Bueno-Marí, R. (2018) Advances in Diagnosis, Surveillance, and Monitoring of Zika Virus: An Update. *Front. Microbiol.* 8:2677. doi: 10.3389/fmicb.2017.02677.eCollection 2017.

[26] Centers for Disease Control and Prevention (CDC), Diagnostic Tests for Zika Virus, *CDC.* https://www.cdc.gov/zika/hc-providers/types-of-tests.html, Accessed on 29 October 2018.

[27] Rodolphe Hamel, R. et al. (2015) Biology of Zika Virus Infection in Human Skin Cells, *J Virol.* 2015 Sep 1; 89(17): 8880–8896; DOI: 10.1128/JVI.00354-15.

[28] Meertens, L. et al. (2017) Axl Mediates ZIKA Virus Entry in Human Glial Cells and Modulates Innate Immune Responses. *Cell Reports,* 18: 324–333.

[29] Delvecchio, R. et al. (2017) Chloroquine, an Endocytosis Blocking Agent, Inhibits Zika Virus Infection in Different Cell Models, *Viruse*s, 8: 322; doi:10.3390/v812.

[30] Stephanie L. Cumberworth, S. L. et al. (2017) Zika virus tropism and interactions in myelinating neural cell cultures: CNS cells and myelin are preferentially affected. *Acta Neuropathol. Commun.,* 5: 50. Published online 2017 Jun 23. doi: [10.1186/s40478-017-0450-8].

[31] Richarda, A. S. et al. (2017). AXL-dependent infection of human fetal endothelial cells distinguishes Zika virus from other pathogenic flaviviruses . *Proc Natl Acad Sci U S A.* 2017 Feb 21;114(8):2024-2029. doi: 10.1073/pnas.1620558114. Epub 2017 Feb 6.

[32] Suan-Sin Foo, S. et al. (2018). Biomarkers and immunoprofiles associated with fetal abnormalities of ZIKV-positive pregnancies, *JCI*

Insight. 2018;3(21):e124152. https://doi.org/10.1172/jci.insight.124152.
[33] Pharmaceutical Research and Manufacturers of America. Biopharmaceutical Research Industry Profile. 2014; Available from: http://www.phrma.org/sites/default/files/pdf/2014_PhRMA_PROFILE.pdf. Accessed December 1, 2014.
[34] Paul, S. M., et al. (2010) How to improve R&D productivity: the pharmaceutical industry's grand challenge. *Nat Rev Drug Discov.* 2010;9(3):203–214.
[35] Pascoalino, B. S. et al. (2016) Zika antiviral chemotherapy: identification of drugs and promising starting points for drug discovery from an FDA-approved library. *F1000 Research* 5:2523, https://f1000research.com/articles/5-2523/v1.
[36] Bhattacharjee, A. K. and Basak, S. C. (2016).Spilled Over Emerging Infectious Diseases Necessitate an Accelerated Drug Design and Discovery Program: Some Comments with Special Reference to Chemoinformatics and the Current Zika Virus Crisis, *Current Computer-Aided Drug Design,* 12(4): 251-252.
[37] Bhattacharjee AK (2018) Pharmacophore modeling applied to mosquito-borne diseases. In: Devillers J (Ed), *Computational Design of Chemicals for the Control of Mosquitoes and Their Diseases*, CRC Press, Taylor & Francis Group, Boca Raton, FL, USA, pp. 139-169.

Biographical Sketches

Subhash C. Basak

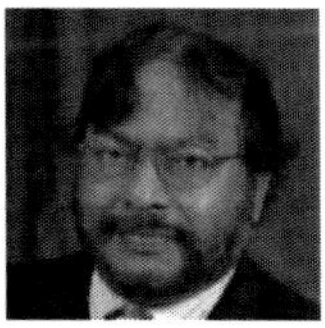

Subhash C. Basak received his PhD in biochemistry in 1981 from the University of Calcutta, India. He was a faculty research Associate in the

Department of Chemistry, University of Minnesota-Duluth, during 1982-1987. Subsequently, during 1987-1911 Basak was a Senior Scientist at the Natural Resources Research Institute (NRRI) and Adjunct Professor in the Department of Chemistry, Biochemistry, and Molecular Biology. He is currently Adjunct Professor in the Department of Chemistry and Biochemistry, University of Minnesota-Duluth. Basak's research areas during the past four decades have been: 1) Biochemistry of psychoactive drugs, 2) Drug tolerance, 3) Structure-activity relationship of drugs and toxicants using mathematical structural descriptors, 4) Development of Novel Topological Indices, 5) Hierarchical QSAR (quantitative structure-activity relationship), 6) Quantitative Molecular Similarity Analysis (QMSA) Methods, 7) Development of novel DNA/ RNA Sequence descriptors and applications, 8) Mathematical Proteomics, 9) Characterization of molecular chirality using Relative Chirality Index (RCI), 10) Modelling in Nanotoxicoproteomics, 11) Characterization of drug addiction, 12) Differential quantitative structure-activity relationship (DiffQSAR) for drug resistance, 13) Statistical methods in QSAR, and 14) Philosophy of mathematical chemistry. He is currently the Editor-in-Chief of the international journal Current Computer Aided Drug Design. He is also past President of the International Society of Mathematical Chemistry.

For details of Basak's publications, please see:

https://www.researchgate.net/profile/Subhash_Basak

Publications from the Last 3 Years:

A) Book:

1) Advances in Mathematical Chemistry and Applications: Volume 1 and 2, 1st Edition

Editors: Subhash Basak Guillermo Restrepo Jose Villaveces

eBook ISBN: 9781681081977

Paperback ISBN: 9781681081984

Bentham Science Publishers and Elsevier

B) Research Papers:

1) Basak, S. C. (2017) The Expanding Landscape of Graph Theoretic Molecular Descriptors: Development, Gradual Diversification of

Descriptor Space, and Applications in QSAR/ QMSA and New Drug Discovery, *Current Computer-Aided Drug Design*, Vol. 13, No. 3, 172-176.

2) Basak, S. C. and Kier, L. B. (2018) Editorial: Current Opioid Overdose Crisis: Some Comments on the Chemicobiological Aspects of Tolerance/Dependence and Abuse Based on Computational Chemistry and Biology, *Current Computer-Aided Drug Design*, 14, No. 3, 175-177.
3) Majumdar, S.; Basak, S.C. (2018) Exploring intrinsic dimensionality of chemical spaces for robust QSAR model development: A comparison of several statistical approaches. *Curr. Comput. Aided Drug Des.*,12(4), 294-301.
4) Majumdar, S. and Basak, S. C. (2018) Beware of External Validation! - A Comparative Study of Several Validation Techniques used in QSAR Modelling, *Current Computer-Aided Drug Design*, 14, in press.
5) Majumdar, S., Basak, S. C., Lungu, C. N., Diudea, M. V. and Grunwald, G. D. (2018) Mathematical structural descriptors and mutagenicity assessment: a study with congeneric and diverse datasets, *SAR and QSAR in Environmental Research*, 29:8, 579-590, DOI: 10.1080/1062936X.2018.1496475
6) Basak, S. C., and S. Majumdar, S. 2016. "Editorial: Chemodescriptor Based QSARs of Structurally Homogeneous Versus Heterogeneous Chemical Data Sets: Some Comments on the Congenericity Principle vis-à-vis Diversity Begets Diversity Principle." *Curr. Comput. Aided Drug Des*. 12: 84-86.
7) Basak, S. C. and Bhattacharjee, A. K. Computational approaches for the design of mosquito repellent chemicals, *Current Medicinal Chemistry*, in press, 2018.
8) Kier, L. B. and Basak, S. C. (2018) Editorial: The Concepts of Pharmacophore/Toxicophores: A Philosophical/Mathematical-cum-Historical Perspective, *Current Computer-Aided Drug Design*, 14, No. 2 103-105.

9) Basak, S. C., Vračko, M. and Witzmann, F. A. (2016) 'Mathematical nanotoxicoproteomics quantitative characterization of effects of multi-walled carbon nanotubes (MWCNT) and TiO2 nanobelts (TiO2−NB) on protein expression patterns in human intestinal cells." *Current Computer-Aided Drug Design*, 12:259-264.
10) Vračko, M., Basak, S. C. and Witzmann, F. A. (2018). Chemometrical analysis of proteomics data obtained from three cell types treated with multi-walled carbon nanotubes and TiO2 nanobelts". *SAR & QSAR in Environmental Research* 29:567-577.
11) Basak, S.C., Nandy, A. (2016) Computer-Assisted Approaches as Decision Support Systems in the Overall Strategy of Combating Emerging Diseases: Some Comments Regarding Drug Design, Vaccinomics, and Genomic Surveillance of the Zika Virus. *Curr. Comp.-Aided Drug Des.* 12(1): 1-3.
12) Nandy, A., Basak, S.C. (2016) Rational design of peptide vaccines against the Zika virus through sequence descriptors: Techniques and Problems. *SOJ Vaccine Res* 1(1): 3.
13) Nandy, A., Basak, S.C. (2016) A Brief Review of Computer-Assisted Approaches to Rational Design of Peptide Vaccines. *Int. J. Mol. Sci.* 17: 666; doi:10.3390/ijms17050666.
14) Nandy, A., Dey, S., Basak, S.C., Bielinska-Waz, D., Waz, P. (2016) Characterizing the Zika Virus Genome – A Bioinformatics Study. *Curr. Comp.-Aided Drug Des* 12: 87-97.
15) Sen D., Dasgupta S., Pal I., Manna S., Basak S.C., Nandy A., Grunwald G. (2016) Intercorrelation of major DNA/RNA sequence descriptors – A preliminary study. *Comp.-Aided Drug Des* 12: 216-228.
16) Nandy, A., Basak, S.C. (2017) Viral epidemics and vaccine preparedness. *J Mol Pathol Epidemiol*. 2: S1-06.
17) Panas, D., Waz, P., Bielinska-Waz, D., Nandy, A., Basak, S.C. (2017) 2D Dynamic Representation of DNA/RNA Sequences as a Characterization Tool of the Zika Virus Genome. *MATCH Commun. Math. Comput. Chem.* 77: 321-332.

18) Dey, S., Nandy, A., Basak, S.C., Nandy, P., Das, S. (2017) A Bioinformatics approach to designing a Zika virus vaccine. *Comput Biol Chem.* 68: 143-152.
19) Nandy, A., Basak, S.C. (2017) Computer-assisted Vaccine Design (CAVD) approach can help in the management of the emerging H7N9 influenza virus. *Curr. Comp.-Aided Drug Des.* 13(3): 264-265. DOI: 10.2174/1573409913041711110160723
20) Nandy, A., Basak, S.C. (2017) The epidemic that shook the world – The Zika virus rampage. *Exploratory Research and Hypothesis in Medicine* 2(3):43–56. doi: 10.14218/ERHM.2017.00018.
21) Dey, S., Roy, P., Nandy, A., Basak, S., Das, S. (2017) Comparison of Base Distributions in Dengue, Zika and Other Flavivirus Envelope and NS5 Genes. In Proceedings of the MOL2NET 2017, International Conference on Multidisciplinary Sciences, 3rd edition, 15 February–20 December 2017; *Sciforum Electronic Conference Series*, Vol. 3. doi:10.3390/mol2net-03-04966
22) Nandy, A., Basak, S. (2017) Some Comments on Mathematical Descriptors of Biomolecular Sequences and their Characteristics. In Proceedings of the MOL2NET 2017, International Conference on Multidisciplinary Sciences, 3rd edition, 15 February–20 December 2017; *Sciforum Electronic Conference Series*, Vol. 3. doi:10.3390/mol2net-03-04967
23) Basak, S., Nandy, A. (2017) A brief account of the search for peptide vaccines. In Proceedings of the MOL2NET 2017, International Conference on Multidisciplinary Sciences, 3rd edition, 15 February–20 December 2017; *Sciforum Electronic Conference Series*, Vol. 3, 2017; doi:10.3390/mol2net-03-05041
24) Panas, D., Waz, P., Bielinska-Waz, D., Nandy, A., Basak, S.C. (2018) An Application of the 2D-Dynamic Representation of DNA/RNA Sequences to the Prediction of Influenza A Virus Subtypes. *MATCH Commun. Math. Comput. Chem.* 80: 295-310.
25) Sen, D., Roy, P., Nandy, A., Basak, S.C., Das, S. (2018) Graphical representation methods: How well do they discriminate between homologous gene sequences? *Chemical Physics* 513: 156-164.

26) Roy, P., Dey, S., Nandy, A., Basak, S.C., Das, S. (2018) Base Distribution in Dengue Nucleotide Sequences Differs Significantly from Other Mosquito-Borne Human-Infecting Flavivirus Members. *Curr Comput Aided Drug Des.* Epub 2018 Jul 30. DOI: 10.2174/1573409914666180731090005.

C) Chapters in Books

1) Basak, S.C.; Majumdar, S. Current landscape of hierarchical QSAR modelling and its applications: Some comments on the importance of mathematical descriptors as well as rigorous statistical methods of model building and validation, In *Advances in Mathematical Chemistry and Applications*; Basak, S. C., Restrepo, G. and Villaveces, J. L. (Eds.), Bentham-Elsevier e-Books, 2016, Vol. 1, pp.251-281.
2) Nandy, A., Basak, S.C. (2018) Bioinformatics in Design of Antiviral Vaccines. Reference Module in Biomedical Sciences. *Encyclopaedia of Biomedical Engineering 2019*, Pages 280-290. https://doi.org/10.1016/B978-0-12-801238-3.10878-5
3) Nandy, A., De, A., Roy, P., Dutta, M., Roy, M., Sen, D., Basak, S.C. (2018) "Alignment-free analyses of nucleic acid sequences using graphical representation (with special reference to pandemic Bird Flu and Swine Flu)", Chapter 9 in S. Singh (ed.), *Synthetic Biology*, https://doi.org/10.1007/978-981-10-8693-9_9, Springer Nature Singapore Pte Ltd.

Apurba K Bhattacharjee

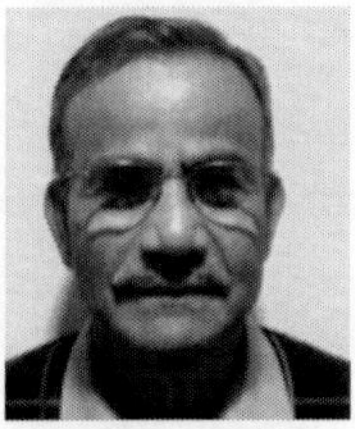

Dr. Apurba K Bhattacharjee is currently an Adjunct Professor at the Department of Microbiology and Immunology at the School of Medicine,

Georgetown University, Washington, DC, U.S.A. Earlier he was a Senior Scientist (Chief Molecular Modeler) at the Walter Reed Army Institute of Research, Maryland, (U.S.A.) from where he retired in 2015. He held a Ph.D. from NEHU, India and a postdoc for three years from the Institute of Topology and Dynamics of Systems (Paris, France) under Professor J.-E. Dubois. Dr. Bhattacharjee has over 30 years of research experience in Computer Assisted Drug Design (CADD), particularly in the application of quantum chemistry, pharmacophore modeling, and virtual screening of compound databases in the discovery of bioactive agents. His background of physical chemistry and quantum chemistry in particular enables him to a deep understanding of different algorithms for specific computations. His focus on Molecular Electrostatic Potentials (MEPs) of bioactive compounds and application of the idea in pharmacophore modeling led him to many successful design and discovery of potential therapeutic agents. His current research interest is in the field of antivirals targeting specifically the dengue and Zika viruses. He has authored and coauthored 130 peer reviewed international publications including several book chapters and five patents.

Publications from the last 3 years:

1) A.K. Bhattacharjee. (2018) Pharmacophore modeling applied to mosquito borne diseases. In "*Computational Design of Chemicals for the Control of Mosquitoes and Their Diseases*" Eds. J. Devillers, Taylor & Francis, *CRC Press*, 139-169.
2) A. Balasubramanian, T. Teramoto, A A. Kulkarni, A.K. Bhattacharjee, R. Padmanabhan. (2017) Antiviral activities of selected antimalarials against dengue virus type and Zika virus. *Antiviral Research* 137: 141-150.
3) A.K. Bhattacharjee, E. Marek, H.T. Le, R. Ratcliffe, J. C. DeMar, D. Pervitsky, R.K. Gordon. (2015) Discovery of non-oxime reactivators using an in silico pharmacophore model of reactivators for DFP-inhibited acetylcholinesterase. *European J. Med. Chem,, 90,* 209-220.
4) M.C. Bagchi, S. Nandi, A.K. Bhattacharjee. (2015) In silico evaluation of 6-(2,6-dichlorophenyl)-pyrido[2,3-d]pyrimidin-7(8H)-

one compounds: an insight into design of less toxic anticancer drugs. Med Chem Res DOI 10.1007/s00044-015-1444-3.

Ashesh Nandy

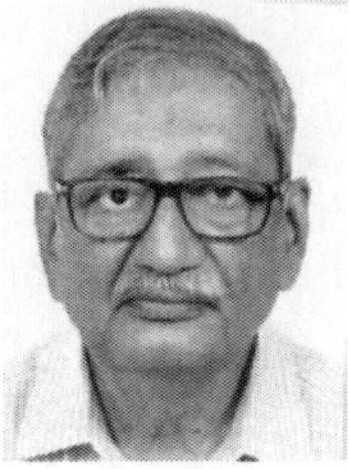

Dr Ashesh Nandy did his PhD in Quantum Electrodynamics in 1971 from the University of California, Santa Barbara, Calif., USA and post-Doc at Syracuse University, Syracuse, New York and Max Planck Institute for Biophysical Chemistry at Göttingen, Germany. Returning to India in 1975, he joined the Indian Association for Cultivation of Science and later the Indian Institute of Chemical Biology. There he developed his model for graphical representation of DNA sequences and pursued the work there and later in Jadavpur University. In 2005-6 he worked on a project at the Natural Resources Research Institute, Duluth, Minnesota, USA developing his approach to designing vaccines for viral diseases using graphical and mathematical models on viral sequences which continues to this day. He has published numerous papers in national and international peer reviewed journals and written several book chapters.

Publications from the Last 3 Years:

1) Basak, S.C., Nandy, A.(2016) Computer-Assisted Approaches as Decision Support Systems in the Overall Strategy of Combating Emerging Diseases: Some Comments Regarding Drug Design, Vaccinomics, and Genomic Surveillance of the Zika Virus. *Curr. Comp.-Aided Drug Des.* 12(1): 1-3.
2) De, A., Sarkar, T., Nandy, A. (2016) Bioinformatics studies of Influenza A hemagglutinin sequence data indicate recombination-like

events leading to segment exchanges. *BMC Res Notes* 9:222. doi 10.1186/s13104-016-2017-3.

3) Nandy, A., Basak, S.C. (2016) Rational design of peptide vaccines against the Zika virus through sequence descriptors: Techniques and Problems. *SOJ Vaccine Res* 1(1): 3.
4) Nandy, A., Basak, S.C. (2016) A Brief Review of Computer-Assisted Approaches to Rational Design of Peptide Vaccines. *Int. J. Mol. Sci.* 17: 666; doi:10.3390/ijms17050666.
5) Dey, S., De, A., Nandy, A. (2016) Rational Design of Peptide Vaccines Against Multiple Types of Human Papillomavirus. *Cancer Informatics* 15(S1): 1-16. doi: 10.4137/CIN.S39071.
6) Nandy, A., Dey, S., Basak, S.C., Bielinska-Waz, D., Waz, P. (2016) Characterizing the Zika Virus Genome – A Bioinformatics Study. *Curr. Comp.-Aided Drug Des* 12: 87-97.
7) Dey, S., Nandy, P., Das, S., Nandy, A. (2016) Comparative Study of Envelope Proteins of Dengue Virus of All Four Serotypes Isolated In India. *J Bioinfo Proteomics Rev* 2(2): 1- 10. doi: 10.15436/2381-0793.16.933.
8) Sen D., Dasgupta S., Pal I., Manna S., Basak S.C., Nandy A., Grunwald G. (2016) Intercorrelation of major DNA/RNA sequence descriptors – A preliminary study. *Comp.-Aided Drug Des* 12: 216-228.
9) Nandy, A., Basak, S.C. (2017) Viral epidemics and vaccine preparedness. *J Mol Pathol Epidemiol.* 2: S1-06.
10) Panas, D., Waz, P., Bielinska-Waz, D., Nandy, A., Basak, S.C. (2017) 2D Dynamic Representation of DNA/RNA Sequences as a Characterization Tool of the Zika Virus Genome. *MATCH Commun. Math. Comput. Chem.* 77: 321-332.
11) Dey, S., Nandy, A., Basak, S.C., Nandy, P., Das, S. (2017) A Bioinformatics approach to designing a Zika virus vaccine. *Comput Biol Chem.* 68: 143-152.
12) Nandy, A., Basak, S.C.(2017) Computer-assisted Vaccine Design (CAVD) approach can help in the management of the emerging H7N9 influenza virus. *Curr. Comp.-Aided Drug Des.* 13(3): 264-265. DOI: 10.2174/1573409913041711110160723

13) Nandy, A., Basak, S.C. (2017) The epidemic that shook the world – The Zika virus rampage. *Exploratory Research and Hypothesis in Medicine* 2(3):43–56. doi: 10.14218/ERHM.2017.00018.
14) Dey, S., Roy, P., Nandy, A., Basak, S., Das, S. (2017) Comparison of Base Distributions in Dengue, Zika and Other Flavivirus Envelope and NS5 Genes. In *Proceedings of the MOL2NET 2017, International Conference on Multidisciplinary Sciences, 3rd edition, 15 February–20 December 2017; Sciforum Electronic Conference Series*, Vol. 3. doi:10.3390/mol2net-03-04966
15) Nandy, A., Basak, S. (2017) Some Comments on Mathematical Descriptors of Biomolecular Sequences and their Characteristics. In Proceedings of the MOL2NET 2017, *International Conference on Multidisciplinary Sciences, 3rd edition, 15 February–20 December 2017; Sciforum Electronic Conference Series, Vol. 3.* doi:10.3390/mol2net-03-04967
16) Basak, S., Nandy, A.(2017) A brief account of the search for peptide vaccines . In *Proceedings of the MOL2NET 2017, International Conference on Multidisciplinary Sciences, 3rd edition, 15 February–20 December 2017; Sciforum Electronic Conference Series, Vol. 3, 2017;* doi:10.3390/mol2net-03-05041
17) Dey, S., Nandy, A., Nandy, P., Das, S. (2018) 'Bioinformatic analysis of envelope gene of the dengue type 3 prevalent in India from 2005 onwards and comparison with dengue type 1', *Int. J. Bioinformatics Research and Applications*, 14(4):357–375.
18) Panas, D., Waz, P., Bielinska-Waz, D., Nandy, A., Basak, S.C. (2018) An Application of the 2D-Dynamic Representation of DNA/RNA Sequences to the Prediction of Influenza A Virus Subtypes. *MATCH Commun. Math. Comput. Chem.* 80: 295-310.
19) Roy, P., Nandy, A. (2018) Nipah virus – An epidemic in the making and a vaccine strategy, *J. Bacteriology and Vaccine Research* 1(1):1004.
20) Sen, D., Roy, P., Nandy, A., Basak, S.C., Das, S. (2018) Graphical representation methods: How well do they discriminate between homologous gene sequences? *Chemical Physics* 513: 156-164.

21) Roy, P., Dey, S., Nandy, A., Basak, S.C., Das, S. (2018) Base Distribution in Dengue Nucleotide Sequences Differs Significantly from Other Mosquito-Borne Human-Infecting Flavivirus Members. *Curr Comput Aided Drug Des.* Epub 2018 Jul 30. DOI: 10.2174/1573409914666180731090005.

Chapters in Books

1) Nandy, A., Basak, S.C. (2018) Bioinformatics in Design of Antiviral Vaccines. Reference Module in Biomedical Sciences. Encyclopedia of Biomedical Engineering 2019, Pages 280-290. https://doi.org/10.1016/B978-0-12-801238-3.10878-5
2) Nandy, A., De, A., Roy, P., Dutta, M., Roy, M., Sen, D., Basak, S.C. (2018) "Alignment-free analyses of nucleic acid sequences using graphical representation (with special reference to pandemic Bird Flu and Swine Flu)", Chapter 9 in S. Singh (ed.), Synthetic Biology, https://doi.org/10.1007/978-981-10-8693-9_9, Springer Nature Singapore Pte Ltd.

In: Zika Virus Surveillance ...
Editors: Subhash C. Basak et al. ISBN: 978-1-53614-970-8

Chapter 2

DISCOVERY OF ANTI-ZIKA DRUGS USING *IN SILICO* PHARMACOPHORE MODELING

Apurba K. Bhattacharjee**, PhD
Biomedical Graduate Research Organization,
Department of Microbiology and Immunology,
School of Medicine, Georgetown University, Washington, DC, US

ABSTRACT

Mosquito borne diseases have overwhelming impacts on public health all over the world with most sufferings in the tropical and subtropical countries. The diseases include malaria, dengue (DENV), Zika (ZIKV), Rift Valley fever, yellow fever, chikungunya (CHKV), West Nile (WNV), Lymphatic filariasis, and Japanese encephalitis. Despite many efforts by WHO and the Bill & Melinda Gates Foundation to combat and eradicate these diseases, mosquito borne infections remain a major problem to the world. Although mosquito repellents are effective and good countermeasures against these infections, issues related to toxicity and resistance limit their protective use. Therapeutic interventions often become necessary for treatment of these infections. Recent outbreak of

* Corresponding Author E-mail: ab3094@georgetown.edu.

Zika virus (ZIKV) in Brazil and quickly spreading to the neighboring countries resulted in a pandemic situation. Since neither any vaccine nor any drug currently available to treat the infection, an urgent necessity is required for both of them. This chapter will deal with *in silico* molecular modeling studies specifically focusing on pharmacophore modeling as tool for rapid identification of compounds as potential therapeutics against ZIKV. In pursuit of the goal, a comprehensive search of literature including author's own research is presented and discussed here.

Keywords: anti-Zika drug discovery, *in silico* modeling, pharmacophores, stereoelectronic profiles, virtual screening, compound databases

INTRODUCTION

Zika virus (ZIKV) like dengue and West Nile belongs to the flavivirus family of viruses transmitted by mosquitos. It was first isolated in 1947 in Uganda, Africa from a sentinel Rhesus macaque and subsequently found in *Aedes africanus* mosquitoes [1]. For further details about the species, refer to Chapter 1 of the book. ZIKV remained less significant than the other major tropical diseases, malaria and dengue, because the original ZIKV infection was known to be a mild febrile illness [2]. However, the scenario rapidly changed due to a series of outbreaks in the Pacific islands [3-6] followed by an explosive emergence in the Americas leading to a pandemic situation [7, 8] in 2014 and 2015. As a result, the WHO had to declare ZIKV outbreak as an international Public Health Emergency. More importantly, it turned into a serious issue due to babies born from ZIKV infected mothers showed microcephaly and neurological complications [8, 9]. Soon the viral infection became a potential threat having profound neurological consequences for normal development of brain to a vast population. Spread of ZIKV from a limited geographical area to different parts of the world has been mostly attributed to increased international travels, globalization of trade, rapid urbanization, poor sanitation, inadequate health services, failure of mosquito control programs due to restrictions on the use of DDT, and insecticide resistance [10]. *Aedes aegypti* and *Ae. albopictus* are the two species of mosquitos primarily responsible for ZIKV transmission [11].

ZIKV-infected adults are also often found to have Guillain-Barre syndrome [2, 12]. Being a member of flavivirus family, ZIKV includes four serotypes of dengue virus (DENV1-4), and West Nile Virus (WNV). It is highly cross-reactive with DENV antibodies and can enhance ZIKV infection with its pathogenesis. All these viruses are re-emerging pathogens due to increased frequency and severity of recent epidemics [13, 14]. The molecular biology and pathogenesis of flaviviruses indicate that their RNA contains a single ORF (open reading frame), translated into a polyprotein, and processed to yield three structural (C, prM & E) and seven nonstructural (NS) proteins from NS1 to NS5 [15]. NS proteins of flavivirus thus play an essential role in polyprotein processing and viral replication [16-20]. The NS5 protein of ZIKV is a specific RNA dependent RNA polymerase (RdRp) which is responsible for the viral genome replication. Further details on NS proteins have been discussed in Chapter 1. Structural elucidation of ZIKV proteins reported recently by proteomic studies could be helpful for structure-based design of anti-ZIKV compounds [21]. Since there are limited *in silico* and etiological studies on ZIKV and non-availability of a detailed compendium of whole genome sequence, the above functional information of proteins, genes, and structural contents should be useful [21]. However, since no vaccine or drug to prevent or treat the infection is known so far, counter measures are urgently necessary.

The goal of the present chapter is to deal with discovery of anti-ZIKV compounds focusing specifically on *in silico* pharmacophore modeling to illustrate how information from three-dimensional structure of small molecules can be utilized for identification and design of new compounds having the potential to counter the infection.

Many *in silico* efforts were used to find potential therapeutics against mosquito borne diseases [22] but pharmacophore modeling is found to be mostly associated with discovery of compounds against cancer, diabetes, and HIV [23]. In the past, combinatorial chemistry coupled with high-throughput screening played important roles in most drug discovery programs. However, in recent years due to large-scale genome mappings and determination of protein structures, a paradigm shift has occurred towards crystallographic structure-based approaches in drug discovery. The shift has led to open new chapters for drug discovery starting from x-ray crystallographic protein structure determination, active site analysis to design and identification of new ligands through virtual screening of databases, docking of ligands at the active site and pharmacophore modeling. Pharmacophores from biologically active ligands have an additional advantage for success even when crystallographic protein structures are unknown [23]. Pharmacophores not only provide useful templates for virtual screening to identify new compounds from databases but also provide useful insights for designing novel ligands and complementary binding features at the active site of an unknown target structure. However, a combined expertise of structure-based knowledge, molecular biology, computational chemistry, docking, pharmacophore modeling, virtual screening, and medicinal chemistry appeared to be most successful in all drug discovery programs.

In silico or computer-assisted molecular modeling (CAMM) has made remarkable advances in recent years for both mechanistic drug design and discovery programs [24–26]. The *in silico* techniques can provide five major types of information for design and discovery of therapeutic agents. These are: (1) three-dimensional structure of a molecule, (2) chemical and physical characteristics of a molecule, (3) comparison of structure of one molecule with the other, (4) graphical visualization of complexes formed between drug-protein or different ligands, and (5) predictions about how related molecules match with the new ones along with an estimate of activity.

Advent of high speed modern computers, astronomical memory and graphic tools have brought new dimensions to computing power by accomplishing computations and visualization of large bio-molecules including simulations of proteins in real time with much greater precision. The graphic tools have not only made visualization for three-dimensional structure of large proteins possible but also made interactive virtual docking experiments between a potential drug-molecule in its binding site a reality. *In silico* methods are now integral part of any basic science research requiring molecular level information. They are routinely used as decision support tools avoiding expensive direct experiments. The advances in *in silico* techniques now allow accurate *ab initio* quantum chemical calculations of stereoelectronic properties, three-dimensional pharmacophore generation, docking and virtual screening to identify potential bioactive compounds [27].

Drug discovery is a complex process with ever changing technologies. It takes almost 10–15 years for transforming a newly discovered molecule from the bench of discovery to a pharmacy for human use. The process has to go through several rounds animal testing, toxicity evaluations and human clinical trials prior to approval by the FDA costing approximately two billion US dollars. Thus, any technology that can improve the efficiency of the process is highly valuable for the pharmaceutical industry [28a]. *In silico* technologies emerged in this way and have proven remarkable success in the past few decades particularly in the domain of intelligent virtual screening of compound databases for identification potential new drugs. The methods are becoming more efficient, precise, reliable and cost effective. Although no model is totally perfect regardless of whatever it represents, virtual screening of hundreds of thousands of compounds in a short time and simulations with three-dimensional protein structures have pushed the technologies to a cutting edge of drug discovery programs [23, 28b, 29].

It is fundamental to understand how a molecule becomes a drug molecule. The concept of lock and key mechanism is the basis of the idea. Thus, when a molecule can optimally bind to the active site of a protein or enzyme involved in a disease to trigger or inhibit its biological response, it can become a potential drug for that disease [30-32]. This is also the basis of the pharmacophore concept. Therefore, at the molecular level, the stereoelectronic properties of the potential drug molecule must optimally interact with the active site of the receptor molecule (protein or enzyme) to trigger or inhibit the specific biological response. Thus, the ability of a bioactive molecule to interact with the complementary active site of a protein or enzyme can be considered as a combination of steric and electronic properties of the molecule. Therefore, study of stereoelectronic properties of bioactive molecules should provide valuable information for understanding the intrinsic "interaction pharmacophore" necessary to find a drug for a disease [26]. This information should also provide a basis for generating a robust statistical pharmacophore model for the potential drug molecule. Once a reliable model is generated, it can enable further design, synthesis and serve as a template for virtual screening of databases to discover more of novel compounds. Since Quantum Chemical (QM) methods provide accurate estimate of stereoelectronic properties, these are frequently used for assessing interaction abilities of potential therapeutic molecules. The profiles generated from stereoelectronic properties are known as the "interaction pharmacophores profiles" [26].

Concept of Pharmacophore

Concept of pharmacophore is critical for understanding the interaction between a receptor and its drug molecule. Paul Ehrlich was first to provide a definition of pharmacophore in early 1900s as "a molecular framework which does carry (*phoros*) the essential features responsible for a drug's (*pharmacon*) biological activity" [30]. Almost hundred years later, Lemont Kier [31a] from molecular orbital theory and Peter Gund [31b] from molecular structural features, provided a similar definition as "a set of structural features in a molecule that is recognized by a receptor and responsible for that molecule's biological activity." Peter Gund is also instrumental for developing the pattern searching method based on functional features (pharmacophores) and used it for identification of new compounds from database searches. He also developed the first software, Molpad for 3D searching [31b]. However, the International Union of Pure and Applied Chemistry (IUPAC) in 1998 provided an official definition of pharmacophore [32]. The definition states that a pharmacophore is "an ensemble of steric and electronic features that are necessary for optimal interaction with a specific receptor target structure (a protein or an enzyme) to trigger or inhibit its biological response" [33]. Although pharmacophore definition indicates an abstract idea, it is possible to represent a pharmacophore in three dimensional space as the statistical distribution of chemical features such as hydrogen bond acceptors & donors, aliphatic & aromatic hydrophobic sites, ring aromaticity, and ionizable sites required for interaction with complementary sites of the target structure. Features of a pharmacophore are represented as vectors and geometrical spheres. The vector directionality features, namely those associated with the hydrogen bonding is derived from symmetry, number of localized lone pairs, and the environment around the atom in a molecule (ligand atom) [33]. More importantly, the concept of pharmacophore leads to the idea that if two structurally different compounds share a similar pharmacophore, the compounds should have similar biological activity. For example, the following illustration (Figure 1) shows two structurally different compounds sharing similar pharmacophore features containing two hydrogen bond acceptors and two hydrophobic sites. Since this pharmacophore was generated as a model for antimalarial activity, both the compounds should have antimalarial activity. Indeed, as predicted, both the compounds showed antimalarial activity [34].

However, pharmacophore is often misrepresented by medicinal chemists [32] because it does not represent any molecule or functional group, it essentially provides an estimate of common molecular interaction capabilities of a set of bioactive compounds for its target structure. The idea is commonly used in drug discovery programs to support medicinal chemists for hit identifications and lead optimizations. Since the pharmacophore idea transcends a chemical structural class and captures only the features responsible for activity, it is very useful for virtual screening of compound databases to identify potentially new active compounds of different chemical classes (chemo-types). Furthermore, it is also be useful for *de novo* design by joining the disjointed chemical features with functional groups to create novel potentially active compounds.

Several ways pharmacophores are derived such as, (a) by analogy to a natural substrate, (b) from known ligands, (c) by inference from a series of dissimilar active analogs, and (d) by direct analysis of the structure of a target protein [32, 35, 36]. However, it is mainly used in two ways to discover potentially active new compounds. In the first approach, *de novo* design by linking the disjointed features of the pharmacophore with chemical fragments to generate a hypothetical structure that is chemically viable and novel. In the second approach, the model can be used as a template for searching compound databases to identify potentially active compounds. The key advantage of virtual screening of database over the *de novo* design is that it allows identification of existing compounds that are either readily available for *in vitro* testing or have a known synthetic procedure for further studies [37].

However, if three-dimensional structure of a target protein or the enzyme is available, small molecule docking procedures can be adopted to perform structure-based virtual screening for identification of an ideal ligand which can be further short listed through pharmacophore modeling. Pharmacophores can also be developed for other molecular properties, such as the ADME (absorption, distribution, metabolism and excretion) properties, toxicity data, lipophilicity, and drug-related properties. Pharmacophore based identification of new active compounds has shown remarkable success in recent years [38-44].

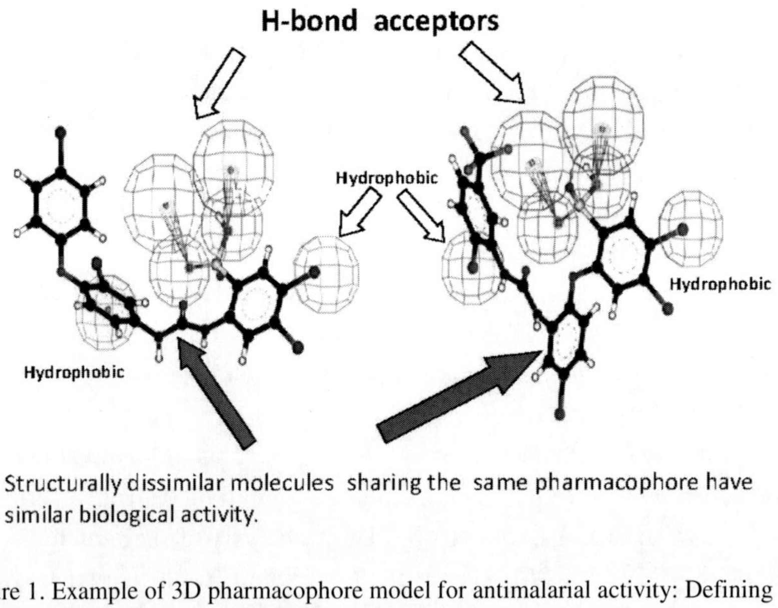

Figure 1. Example of 3D pharmacophore model for antimalarial activity: Defining feature requirements on two dissimilar molecular structures.

However, a few implicit assumptions of pharmacophore models are important to keep in mind [23]. Model generation from a set of active compounds, its validation and database searches using a pharmacophore assumes the following:

a) the structures used in developing the pharmacophore are responsible for the biological activity, not their metabolites,
b) the conformation of a structure mapping the model is its bioactive conformation,
c) the binding site is the same for all molecules in the proposed model,
d) biological activity is accounted only in terms of thermodynamic equilibrium, particularly by enthalpy energy considerations, assuming entropy for the molecules to be similar,
e) kinetics of molecular transformation are ignored, and
f) transport properties, diffusion and solvent effects too are avoided.

Regardless of the above assumptions, pharmacophore is a very important effective tool for medicinal chemists in drug discovery programs. Generation of virtual libraries and screening by pharmacophores have become a routine task in drug discovery research. Basic concept of mapping pharmacophore features on functional groups of screened compounds has not only allowed identification of a variety of compounds, the models themselves are useful as great visualization tools. For example, a rotatable 3D pharmacophore model mapped on a protein-ligand complex can provide useful insights about interactions and therefore can facilitate interdisciplinary discussions with medicinal chemists, synthetic chemists, toxicologists, and pharmacologists for a successful drug discovery approach [44]. However, experimental validation of identified compounds will be necessary to establish the true reliability of the generated model.

IMPORTANCE OF PHARMACOPHORE MODELING IN DRUG DISCOVERY

As mentioned earlier, discovery and development of new therapeutics are expensive and complex processes with ever changing technologies. *In silico* or virtual screening techniques successfully emerged during the past few decades as efficient tools to support drug discovery programs cost effectively [45, 46]. However, use of pharmacophore for virtual screening of databases became quite an intelligent knowledge based tool to support discovery of new class of compounds as potential drug molecules. The process serve as a complimentary tool to high-throughput screening (HTS) for rapid and effective experimental assay for a large pool of compounds. Since screening for compounds by pharmacophore is essentially a knowledge-based approach, it implicitly provides certain information about the nature of the receptor-binding site or the nature of the ligand expected to bind effectively at the active site. However, the type of procedure followed in virtual screening for compound databases rely upon availability of information as input and requirement for the output [45, 46].

Pharmacophore models significantly contributed to the discovery of drugs in recent the past along with retrieving inhibitors for various drug targets [39-43].

METHODS FOR PHARMACOPHORE MODEL GENERATION

Pharmacophore models can be generated using pharmacophore generation methods. Two widely used pharmacophore modeling and screening software programs are LigandScout [47] and Discovery Studio [48]. These methods are used for generation, validation, and application for virtual screening of compound databases to identify new compounds. The 3D QSAR pharmacophore generation protocol utilizes the Discovery Studio [48] or an earlier version of the software known as CATALYST HypoGen algorithm [49] to derive structure-activity relationship (SAR) hypothesis from a set of ligands with known activity values. Input ligand data should contain two properties: activity and uncertainty factors associated with reproducibility of the activities. Briefly, the methodology allows the use of known structure and activity data from a set of compounds (known as training set) to create a hypothesis (pharmacophore) which characterizes the activity of the training set. The uncertainty factor represents a ratio range of uncertainty in activity values based on an expected statistical dispersion of biological data collections. Thus, an uncertainty value of 3 (or lower if the reproducibility of experimental data is more accurate) means that the actual activity of a particular compound is assumed to be situated somewhere ranging from one-third to three times of the reported activity value of that compound. Thus, for example, an experimental value of 15.0 mM (EC_{50} or IC_{50}) will cover a range of 5.0 to 45.0 mM (EC_{50} or IC_{50}) for the given uncertainty value of 3 for generation of the pharmacophore model. Many parameters are required to be tested. The pharmacophore model itself can be used as a template for database searches [50]. Conformational models of known structures are generated by creating a training set of compounds that emphasizes representative coverage within a range of the permissible Boltzmann population with significant abundance (within10.0 kcal/mol) of the calculated global minimum. This conformational model for pharmacophore generation that aims to identify the best three-dimensional arrangement of chemical features is usually selected for the modeling study. The pharmacophore features such as hydrogen bond donor/acceptor, hydrophobic sites and positively or negatively charged ionizable sites distributed over a three dimensional space describe the activity variations among the training set.

The chemical features selected are usually the followings: Hydrogen bond acceptor (HBA): 2 to 4, hydrogen bond donor (HBD): 0 to 2, hydrophobic (HY): 1 to 3, and ring aromatic (RA): 0 to 1. The minimum inter-feature distance is 3 which specifies the minimum spacing of 3Å between feature points. The mapping of a pharmacophore model onto an active compound is determined by a "fit score."

The fit score is:

$$Fit = \sum w \left(1 - \sum (Disp/Tol)^2\right)$$

where the equation variables are:

- w = adaptively determined weight of the hypothesis function based on dispersion and tolerance of the feature from the centroid.
- The fit score does not only check the feature's mapping but also contains a distance term that measures the distance between the

feature on the molecule to the centroid of the feature. Both terms are used to calculate the geometric fit value.

The quality of a pharmacophore model is evaluated by the following set of parameters: (a) correlation value, (b) total cost, (c) null cost, (d) fixed cost and (e) statistical data. To get a reliable pharmacophore model, the total cost should be significantly different from the null cost. For a pharmacophore hypothesis, a value of 40-60 bits between total cost and null cost (difference between the costs) might indicate that it had 75-90% possibility of correlating the data. Greater the value of the cost difference, less likely that the pharmacophore will reflect a chance correlation [48, 49].

PHARMACOPHORE VALIDATION

Validation of a quantitative pharmacophore model is extremely important for reliability of the model. It is usually assessed from the model's ability to identify active compounds and accuracy in activity predictions. In addition, a test set of compounds is constructed to determine the correlation (R^2) with the generated pharmacophore and comparing it with that of the training set. Furthermore, Fischer's validation [48, 49] and decoy sets are employed to validate the generated model. To achieve 95% confidence level of a model, the Fischer's randomization is conducted by scrambling activity data of the training set of compounds, assigning them new values, and then generating pharmacophores using the same features and parameters originated from the first pharmacophore. The significance of pharmacophores is to be calculated using the following formula: $[1 - (1 + X) / Y] \times 100\%$, where X and Y are the number of training and test set molecules. Scramble runs are important to prove that the pharmacophore model was not generated by a chance correlation but based on meaningful correlations [48, 49]. However, for ultimate validation of the pharmacophore, compounds identified are to be experimentally tested, first through *in vitro* tests and subsequently through *in vivo* testing if the compounds are found promising in *in vitro* tests [50].

VIRTUAL SCREENING OF COMPOUND DATABASES USING GENERATED PHARMACOPHORE MODEL

For identification of potentially active compounds, the most reliable pharmacophore model is employed as a search query for virtual screening of compound databases. By the most reliable pharmacophore model, it means to have the highest confidence level of all generated models. Mapping the model onto the most potent compound of the training set could be the starting template for searches. However, for a better efficiency of the search, converting the mapped model of the most potent compound to a 3D shape based template will serve better because it will reflect the complementarity of steric volume associated with the active site in the target structure. Both pharmacophore features and steric requirements will together then be embedded in the screening procedure [51]. Successful searches of databases from both trial and test sets along with "goodness of hits" (GH) are identified by using the following equation,

$$GH = \{Ha\ (3A+Ht)/4HtA\} \times \{1-Ht-Ha/D-A\} \ ....$$

"Ht" is the total number of trial compounds, "Ha" is number of known active compounds in the test database, "A" is the number of active compounds in the database, "D" is the total number of compounds in the database [33, 48, 49]. The identified compounds are to be mapped onto the pharmacophore model and their predicted activities, EC_{50} or IC_{50} values are to be noted. Compounds with predicted activity less than 500nM are usually tested for *in vitro* (experimental) activity [50].

BIOLOGICAL ASSAY

It is important to note that although pharmacophore based search of compound databases is an efficient tool for extracting potential bioactive compounds, it is necessary to experimentally test the identified compounds and iteratively refine the model. Thus, developing an appropriate biological assay for testing compounds is an important component of the pharmacophore based drug discovery process. Compounds that map well onto the best generated pharmacophore model showing estimated activities EC_{50} or IC_{50} values less than 500nM are usually considered for *in vitro* evaluations.

To evaluate the anti-ZIKV activities of identified compounds, plaque assays can be used. In our laboratory, ZIKV virus (MR766) at MOI 1 was used for evaluation [52]. Vero cells were used for collection of supernatants from ZIKV-infected and drug-treated cells as well as control ZIKV infected cells without drugs. Plaque assays were set up in 24-well plates that were seeded with Vero cells following a protocol as described in Section 2.4 of the publication [52]. Based on the promise of *in vitro* evaluations, favorable drug-like properties and *in silico* ADME/Toxicity assessments, the identified compounds may be short-listed for *in vivo* studies [50].

Pharmacophore Modeling for Discovery of Potential Therapeutics against Zika Virus

Pharmacophore modeling and *in silico* studies used for potential discovery of therapeutics against ZIKV from published literature are discussed in this section. However, no therapeutic compound against ZIKV found solely from pharmacophore modeling-3D QSAR study was reported in the published literature so far. Thus, other reported *in silico* studies are discussed in length for a possible future scope for pharmacophore modeling in the pursuit of new anti-ZIKV therapeutics.

Although no pharmacophore modeling study to identify new anti-ZIKV compounds was performed, several antimalarial chloroquine analogues including chloroquine and its derivatives were reported to exhibit ant-ZIKV activity in Vero cells and in human brain microvascular endothelial along with neutral stem cells [53]. Structural modifications, particularly at the C-4 position of N-(2-arylmethylimino)ethyl-7-chloroquinolin-4-amine derivatives was reported to show more potent anti-ZIKV activity than chloroquine [54]. Since pharmacophore models for chloroquine and related analogues are known [55-57], there could be a possible scope for utilizing the antimalarial pharmacophore model for virtual screening of databases to identify new potential anti-ZIKV compounds. In pursuit this objective, we recently reported [52] an *in silico* modeling study on twelve antimalarial aminoquinoline derivatives by developing an "interaction pharmacophore model" from quantum chemically (QC) calculated stereoelectronic properties of the compounds. Similarity analysis of the "interaction pharmacophore model" with other published aminoquinoline derivatives from literature [58-60] and comparing with our model, we identified three antimalarial aminoquinolines, Quinacrine (QC), Mefloquine (MQ), and GSK369796 (Figure 2a) for testing against ZIKV in *in vitro* assay developed in our laboratory [52].

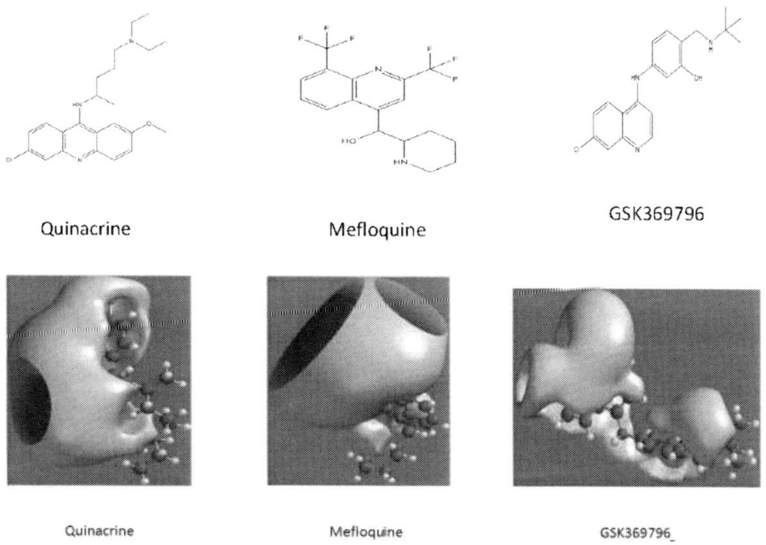

Figure 2. (a) Chemical structure of the three anti-ZIKV compounds, quinacrine, mefloquine and GSK369796. (b) Molecular Electrostatic Potential isosurfaces of quinacrine, mefloquine, and GSK369796 extending beyond the van der Waals surface of each molecule at –20.9 kJ/mol.

Experimental analysis of the three aminoquinolines indicated all three to have potent activity against ZIKV, EC_{50} values: 2.27 ± 0.14 mM (for QC); 3.95 ± 0.21 mM (for MQ); and 2.57 ± 0.09 mM (for GSK369796) [52]. Inspection of interaction pharmacophore profiles of the three compounds (Figure 2b) indicates a large extended negative potential region over the N atom containing aromatic ring in the compounds. Quinacrine (QC), mefloquine (MQ) and GSK369796 (to a smaller extent) exhibit unique profiles with a large hole over the N atom in the aromatic ring. The profiles indicate a nucleophilic suction like interaction abilities of the compounds with the complementary electrophilic sites in the receptor. Probably, this unique feature in them is responsible for potent ZIKV activity of the compounds. Thus, the pharmacophore requirements for potent anti-ZIKV activity of the compounds appear to be: a strong H-bond acceptor site, a moderately strong H-bond donor site and a large distribution of hydrophobic area in the molecules. However, further *in silico* and experimental studies on antimalarial compounds are required for consideration of "repurposing" of old antimalarial drugs as potential anti-ZIKV drugs.

Drug repurposing is a well-known strategy for pharmaceutical industries to speed up the discovery process. It is essentially the use of a known FDA approved drug for treatment of a new indication. The advantage of drug repurposing over the traditional drug discovery and development approach is that it is both time and cost effective. Since FDA approved drugs are already in clinical use, clinical trials for a different therapeutic application may likely to be less risky as adverse toxicological study reports, if any are already known. Additionally, drug repurposing can also serve old drug compounds as starting materials for development of leads for new therapeutic purposes. Therefore, repurposing approach for old antimalarial compounds using pharmacophore modeling can be important in the selection process.

Since neglected viral diseases like ZIKV infection, dengue, chikungunya etc. are less likely to get attention from big pharmaceutical industries, repurposing approach for old drugs applying *in silico* modeling could be a quicker strategy in getting drugs to the market for treatment of these infections. Thus, for example, PHA-690509, a cyclin dependent kinase

(CDK) inhibitor is recently reported to have potent anti-ZIKV activity [61] and therefore, study on known CDK inhibitors could be useful for anti-ZIKV therapeutics discovery. Several combinations with CDK inhibitors were shown to have inhibitory caspase-3 activity in SNB-19 cells [61]. It is worthwhile to mention here that our earlier reported malarial CDK (pfmrk) pharmacophore model [35] could be a useful guiding template for virtual screening from a large pool of antimalarial CDK (pfmrk) inhibitors to identify potential anti–ZIKV compounds. The malarial CDK pharmacophore model was developed and validated by us that allowed identification of several new antimalarial CDK inhibitors [35]. Therefore, repurposing attempt for additional CDK inhibitors using *in silico* modeling could be attempted for discovery of potential anti-ZIKV drugs.

Identification of ZIKV antivirals from an FDA-approved library of drugs is already reported to be a promising starting point for repurposing for new drug applications [62]. Pharmacophore modeling could be a very helpful supporting tool for the approach. A pharmacophore-based shortlisting of the approved drugs for *in vitro* testing can be a rapid and efficient approach. From the severity perspectives of ZIKV infection, attempts should not only be confined for discovery of drugs and vaccines, efforts should also be directed toward vector control and palliative care to ease the burden of the infection.

Different approaches and methodologies were attempted in search for agents to counter ZIKV by testing specific compounds with known antiviral activity to screening of compound libraries with hundreds of bioactive molecules. One such reported effort deals with identification of antiviral compounds that include compounds targeting both viral and the cellular components [63]. These researchers tested specific compounds with known antiviral activity in virus models and also compounds from bioactive compound libraries including antivirals already approved for human use. The compounds included nucleosides analogues, nucleoside synthetic inhibitors, targeting viral enzymes, anticancer and anti-inflammatory molecules, antibiotics, and antiparasitics [63]. The study was extensive for understanding biology and mechanism of anti-ZIKV activity of compounds but so far no drug against ZIKV has resulted from the study. Aside, no *in silico* study was performed on the compounds [63]. In addition, data-driven strategies to model and mitigate the threat for ZIKV have aslo been explored. For details of this approach, Chapter 4 may be referred.

Another study emphasizes the need for an alternative strategy over the traditional drug discovery programs and emphasizes structure-based pharmacophore to be a better tool for discovery of anti-ZIKV therapeutics [64]. The researchers observed that structure-based pharmacophore when combined with docking lead to a better outcome than just the pharmacophore-based screening. Challenges for receptor flexibility issues and appropriate pharmacophore model selection from a large pool of generated models were discussed. They concluded that the tools for structure-based pharmacophore discovery are continuing to evolve, and therefore this approach should have wider impact to traditional approaches [64].

In another study, the authors reported antibodies capable of targeting a conformational epitope isolated from dengue patients could potently neutralize ZIKV virus [65]. They found the crystal structure of two of these antibodies in complex with the envelope protein of ZIKV that contained a conserved epitope and the interaction site of the protein dimer as the precursor prM protein during virus maturation. The authors concluded that a comparison of ZIKV and DENV (dengue virus) immunocomplexes should provide the lead for a rational design of epitope-focused broad-spectrum vaccine for combating both viruses simultaneously [65]. For details on immunological discussions on ZIKV Chapter 3 may be referred. Although the study does not deal with any *in silico* aspect, clearly there is a scope for structure-based modeling as the crystal structures of the two immunocomplexes have been established.

By using molecular dynamics (MD) simulations, another study reported the molecular behavior of ZIKV NS3h protein in the presence and absence of single-stranded RNA (ssRNA) with potential implications for NS3h activity and inhibition [66]. The authors suggested that the presence of RNA generates important interactions with the RNA binding loop leading to a stabilization to remain in a closed conformation. The closed conformation should keep the ssRNA bound to the protein for a sufficient time to enable the unwinding/replication activities of NS3h. The authors demonstrated through AutoLigand calculations that conformational changes in the RNA binding loop can change the nature and location for the optimal ligand binding site. The information could be helpful for *in silico* design and discovery of new inhibitors of NS3h as potential anti-ZIKV compounds [66].

In another study, ligand-binding features of ATPase and ssRNA sites of the NS3 helicase were characterized [67]. The authors used FDA approved drugs, such as Ivermectin, Lapachol and HMC-HO1α to demonstrate their inhibitory effects on the ZIKV NS3 helicase enzyme. The pharmacophore features of the drugs were determined to conclude the importance of those features in Lapachol, HMC-HO1α and Ivermectin for designing potent hybrid drugs against co-infections of ZIKV, dengue and chikungunya [67].

Another structural study performed by a Czech group of researchers on selected triphosphate analogs reported discovery of 20-Cmethylated nucleosides showing strong inhibitory activity of RNA-dependent RNA polymerase (RdRp). The authors suggested that traditional 20-Cemethylated nucleosides could be a new brand of scaffolds to counter the ZIKV virus [68].

A recent review [69] summarizes various progress in the design of inhibitors of NS3 protein, small molecules, methyltransferase inhibitors, interferons, repurposed drugs, computer aided design of drugs, neutralizing antibodies, convalescent serum, antibodies that limit antibody-dependent enhancement, and herbal medicines. The review also discusses covalent inhibitors of a viral protein and anti-Toll-like receptor molecules to counter ZIKV associated diseases [69].

Barrows et al. [70] recently published a screening study on FDA-approved drugs in search for inhibitors of ZIKV. Through *in vitro* screening of 774 compounds, twenty compounds were found to reduce ZIKV infection. A few selected from those twenty compounds were further found to inhibit ZIKV infection in human cervical, placental, neural stem cell lines, and primary human amnion cells [70]. Anti-flaviviral drugs such as bortezomib, mycophenolic acid and daptomycin having no previously known anti-ZIKV activity were identified as inhibitors for ZIKV infection

[70]. Overall, the study identified several drugs that may have the potential for further studies including clinical trials for ZIKV. In addition, the study provides a resource of small molecules for *in silico* pharmacophore modeling to further screen the FDA-approved library of drugs for shortlisting potential candidates against ZIKV.

More recently, Ekins et al. provided [71] a successful strategy for discovery of ant-ZIKV compounds identifying five potential drugs through screening of the NIH clinical library of compounds. This clinical library contains 725 chemically diverse FDA-approved drugs with a few known and unknown mechanism of actions. From a primary screening of the library, 22 compounds were reported to have potent anti-ZIKV activity of which five were found promising. Their five shortlisted hits are Lovastatin (Pubchem CID: 53232), 5-Fluorouracil (Pubchem CID: 3385); 6-Azauridine (Pubchem CID: 5901); Palonosetron (Pubchem CID: 6337614) and Kitasamycin (Pubchem CID: 44634697). These FDA-approved drugs were reported to have a wide range of therapeutic applications including hypolipidemic activity, cancer treatments, antineoplastic and antipsoriatic activities, antimetabolite, antagonistic & antiemetic properties, and antibiotic property with antimicrobial efficacy against a variety of pathogens [71]. Since pharmacophore development can transcend chemical structures, pharmacophore modeling on this library of chemically diverse compounds can have the potential for further discovery and design of novel anti-ZIKV compounds.

Another study reported four anti-ZIKV compounds through screening a limited proprietary library of small organic compounds by confirming potent anti-ZIKV activity in *in vitro* plaque assay [72]. The identified compounds described as highly potent bioactive leads, the most active analogs showing activity in low picomolar ranges. The "leads" reported to contain certain common structural features which can be helpful for developing pharmacophore model to design the next generation(s) of anti-ZIKV compounds.

In another recently reported study [73], Ncube et al. found a type of nucleoside adenosine analog, NITD008 to be an antiviral drug. It was developed as a broad spectrum antiviral against several flavivirus infections including dengue, West Nile, yellow fever, Powassan, hepatitis C, Kyasanur Forest disease, Omsk hemorrhagic fever and ZIKV [73]. But due to undesirable toxicity of the compound, no clinical study was reported. However, the researchers explored the binding landscape of the compound in complex with five detrimental *flaviviruses* at the RNA polymerase active sites and generated a pharmacophore model for design of small molecules that may inhibit *flaviviruses* in a broad spectrum manner. They concluded that the pharmacophore approach would provide a robust cornerstone to the medicinal chemists for synthesis of multifunctional inhibitors that will eliminate cross-resistance and toxicity as well as improve patient adherence. However, no specific anti-ZIKV compound was reported through this study [73].

Future Perspectives

Although ZIKV infection was ignored for many decades, past few years saw significant efforts in search for antivirals to counter the infection despite funding shortages [71]. Different approaches and methodologies were adopted ranging from testing specific compounds with known antiviral activity in different virus models to searching hundreds of bioactive compounds from compound libraries including FDA approved drugs for other human uses. The identified compounds were found to target cellular components of the virus. The compounds include nucleoside analogues, synthetic nucleoside inhibitors, viral enzymes, anticancer, anti-inflammatory, antibiotics, and antimalarials. However, selection of compounds remained an important issue since in many instances promising *in vitro* antiviral activity could not be translated into human use [74]. One reason for this failure is stated to be due to the limitation of test assays for immune-deficient mouse models only. The assays were not extended to nonhuman primates [74]. The issue became significant as the target population for anti-ZIKV therapy is found to be primarily the immune deficient people and pregnant women. Therefore, experiments using animals should include additional information, such as time-resolution and measurement of different processes within one single animal to show inter-relationships with mathematical modelling. Furthermore, distinction between a drug and system properties should be available to translate between species along with different conditions. The mathematical models should incorporate all information from animals. Thus, for pharmacophore modeling, caution has to be used while creating training sets of compounds or drugs to incorporate the above conditions including anti-ZIKV activities of immune deficient population and pregnant women before virtual screening of compound libraries to identify new potential anti-ZIKV compounds.

Due to the urgent need for antiviral drugs and vaccines to counter the ZIKV infection, Ekins and co-workers [71] from their vast treasure trove of open source collections and expertise suggested the following six approaches to achieve the goal:

1. To develop a ZIKV cell based *in vitro* assay that would be capable of medium scale to high throughput screening. Since developing such assay requires a special protective laboratory (BSL 2 type lab), it may be difficult for many academic institutions to participate in ZIKV research. However, setting up a plaque assay may be an alternative approach for rapid evaluations of anti-ZIKV activity of compounds as described earlier [52].
2. Second, to test all available FDA approved antiviral drugs in ZIKV validated assays to determine efficacies. Next step would be to shortlist drugs showing promising *in vitro* results for *in vivo* evaluations. However, selection of compounds should be judiciously considered since promising *in vitro* activity may not automatically translate for human use as mentioned earlier and for that reason, adequate steps are necessary as reported [74].
3. To explore and study the genome of ZIKV extensively in order to apply it for a target-based *in silico* chemotherapeutic approach on the FDA approved antiviral drugs, specifically active against the ZIKV prior to *in vitro* testing [75].

4. Although x-ray crystallographic structure for ZIKV is not yet resolved, a three dimensional structure by cryo-electron microscopy (cryo-EM) and image reconstruction for ZIKV is available [52b]. Moreover, the crystal structure of the full-length ZIKV-NS5 protein has been determined with 3.05 A° resolution [76]. This structure is reported to be similar to the NS5 structure of Japanese encephalitis virus protein and suggests opportunities for discovery of broad spectrum antivirals including against ZIKV from this structure-based drug design approach targeting either its MTase or RdRp domain. In addition, homology models for ZIKV may be built from dengue virus crystal structure and target compounds found active against the dengue virus [52] for its known cross-reactivity with anti-DENV antibodies [13, 14].
5. To study and understand the target based mechanism of *in vitro* active (whole cell screening) of compounds identified through earlier *in silico* and *in vitro* approaches for target-activity validation.
6. Finally, to test the promising candidate compounds in animal models of ZIKV infection such as the mouse model and primate models before recommending for clinical trials.

With an established 3D structure of ZIKV protein, discovery for anti ZIKV compounds could be attempted through a combined approach of structure-based drug design, docking of ligands and pharmacophore modeling from known active compounds. All these approaches could be useful for virtual screening of compound databases and helpful for identification of potential new anti-ZIKV candidates. However, it is important to note that even though the 3D structure of ZIKV protein may be perfectly determined, certain specific features, such as the polarization factors and hydrogen bonding effects arising from specific solvation patterns of water molecules in the common ATP-binding pockets and dynamic target-inhibitor interactions occurring intermittently to account for specificity of certain inhibitors may not be available or detectible by crystallography. In order to account for such interactions, *in silico* methods, particularly quantum chemical methods with molecular dynamics could be more useful than most of the experimental methods. In addition, protein/ligand binding affinity predictions from docking results of diverse drug-like molecules using 2D Bayesian categorization procedures may be helpful to build better training sets. Success of this approach has been reported earlier [77]. Moreover, alternative targets for discovery of ZIKV drugs should also be explored. A recent report suggested Axl receptor (a tyrosine kinase) to be a target for ZIKV which functions by inhibiting its dimerization considered to be crucial for virus entry. These researchers experimentally validated the hypothesis by demonstrating anti-ZIKV activities of compounds such as warfarin and a few similar structural analogues identified using *in silico* studies [78]. Thus, there is a scope for further *in silico* studies including pharmacophore modeling targeting the Axl receptor. However, for accomplishing a successful ZIKV drug discovery and development program, the research team should have a good synthetic chemistry support along with expertise from molecular biologists and modeling groups to facilitate a rapid lead optimization.

CONCLUSION

Pharmacophore modeling demonstrates a rational approach for discovery of potential therapeutic candidates solely from structure-activity relationships of known bioactive compounds. However, testing for efficacies of identified compounds, first *in vitro* followed by *in vivo* if found promising is absolutely necessary. Stereoelectronic property analysis of training sets of active compounds can help to generate reliable pharmacophore models. Although a model may be solely from structure-activity relationship study, it should be consistent with observations from X-ray crystal target structure if known. For unknown receptor structures, pharmacophore could be helpful to predict the complimentary interaction capabilities of the target active site. However, it is important to note that despite perfect mapping of a pharmacophore model onto compounds, many short listed compounds may show poor experimental activities. Thus, a pharmacophore directed database search may be an efficient approach for extracting potential bioactive compounds, it is necessary to experimentally test the identified compounds and iteratively refine the model. Perfect mapping of any molecule to the pharmacophore model does not guarantee its experimental activity despite reflecting adequate receptor complementarity. There may be several factors lacking, such as perfect fit to the active site due to steric hindrance, electrostatics, lipophilicity, and other unforeseen parameters. Therefore, all pharmacophore based identified compounds may not have similar biological activities despite reasonably well mapping onto the model. Nevertheless, pharmacophore models are very useful tools for identification of potential therapeutics as seen from various studies. Therefore, application of pharmacophore modeling for discovery of potential new therapeutics against ZIKV may be summarized as follows:

1. Pharmacophore models are useful and efficient tools for drug discovery. Therefore, it should be utilized for discovery of anti-ZIKV compounds.
2. It is important to note that there is no guarantee all the compounds identified using pharmacophore models will show potent activity.
3. Down-selected compounds are to be tested in *in vitro* assays first and subsequently in animals based on the promise of *in vitro* efficacy.
4. Iterative use of 3D shape based pharmacophore searching in conjunction with a large virtual compound library can be very effective for identifying new chemotypes with enhanced *in vitro* activity relative to the target molecule.
5. *In silico* ADME/toxicity evaluations and docking methods could be useful for down selection of compounds.
6. In short, the *in silico* methods can maximize the efficiency for discovery of anti-ZIKV therapeutics.

ACKNOWLEDGMENTS

The author gratefully acknowledges valuable suggestions from numerous colleagues in the department for developing and improving the manuscript. Special thanks to Professor R. Padmanabhan in the department for introducing me to the field of antiviral research targeting dengue and ZIKV viruses.

REFERENCES

[1] Dick GW, Kitchen SF, Haddow AJ (1952) Zika virus. I. Isolations and serological specificity. *Transaction Royal Society of Tropical Medicine and Hygiene* 46(5):509–20. PMID: 12995440.

[2] Petersen LR, Jamieson DJ, Powers AM, Honein MA (2016) Zika virus. *New England Journal Medicine* 374:1552–1563. https://doi.org/10.1056/NEJMra1602113.

[3] Duffy MR, Chen TH, Hancock WT, Powers AM, Kool JL, Lanciotti RS, Pretrick M, Marfel M, Holzbauer S, Dubray C, Guillaumot L, Griggs A, Bel M, Lambert AJ, Laven J, Kosoy O, Panella A, Biggerstaff BJ, Fischer M, Hayes EB (2009) Zika virus outbreak on Yap Island, Federated States of Micronesia. *New England Journal Medicine* 360(24):2536–43. doi: 10.1056/ NEJMoa0805715 PMID: 19516034.

[4] Dupont-Rouzeyrol M, O'Connor O, Calvez E, Daure`s M, John M, Grangeon JP, Gourinat AC (2015) Co-infection with Zika and dengue viruses in 2 patients, New Caledonia, 2014. *Emerging Infectious Diseases* 21: 381–382.

[5] Roth A, Mercier A, Lepers C, Hoy D, Duituturaga S, Benyon E, Guillaumot L, Souares Y (2014). Concurrent outbreaks of dengue, chikungunya and Zika virus infections - an unprecedented epidemic wave of mosquito-borne viruses in the Pacific 2012-2014. *European Surveillance 19*, Published online October 16.

[6] Tognarelli J, Ulloa S, Villagra E, Lagos J, Aguayo C, Fasce R, Parra B, Mora J, Becerra N, Lagos N, Vera L, Olivares B, Vilches M, Fernández J(2016) A report on the outbreak of Zika virus on Easter Island, South Pacific, 2014. *Archives of Virology* 161: 665–668.

[7] Fauci AS, Morens DM (2016) Zika Virus in the Americas–Yet Another Arbovirus Threat. *New England Journal Medicine* 374: 601–604.

[8] Lednicky J., Beau De Rochars VM, El Badry M, Loeb J, Telisma T, Chavannes S, Anilis G, Cella E, Ciccozzi M, Rashid M, Okech B, Salemi M, Morris Jr JG (2016) Zika Virus Outbreak in Haiti in 2014: Molecular and Clinical Data. *PLoS Neglected Tropical Diseases* 10:e0004687. https://doi.org/10.1371/journal.pntd.0004687.

[9] World Health Organization (2016) Zika situation report: Zika virus, microcephaly and Guillain-Barre Syndrome. *WHO.* http://www.who.int/ emergencies/zika-virus/situation-report/7-april-2016/en/. Published April 7, 2016. Accessed September 30, 2016.

[10] Benelli G (2015) Plant-borne ovicides in the fight against mosquito vectors of medical and veterinary importance: a systematic review. *Parasitology Research* 114:3201–3212.

[11] Musso D, Gubler DJ (2016) Zika virus. *Clinical Microbiological Review* 29:487–524. doi: 10.1128/CMR.00072-15).

[12] Fontes CA, Dos Santos AA, Marchiori E (2016) Magnetic resonance imaging findings in Guillain-Barre´ syndrome caused by Zika virus infection. *Neuroradiology*. Published onlinc April 11, 2016.

[13] Lam SK (2013) Challenges in reducing dengue burden; diagnostics, control measures and vaccines. *Expert Review Vaccines* 12:995-1010.

[14] Villar L, Dayan GH, Arredondo-Garcia JL, Rivera DM, Cunha R, Deseda C, Reynales H, Costa MS, Morales-Ramirez JO, Carrasquilla G, Rey LC, Dietze R, Luz K, Rivas E, Miranda Montoya MC, Cortes Supelano M, Zambrano B, Langevin E, Boaz M, Tornieporth N, Saville M, Noriega F, Group CYDS (2015) Efficacy of a tetravalent dengue vaccine in children in Latin America. *New England Journal Medicine* 372:113-123.

[15] Lindenbach D, Thiel HJ, Rice C (2007) Flaviviridae: the viruses and their replication. In: Knipe DM, Howley PM (Eds.). *Field's Virology, 5 ed.* Lippincott-Raven Publishers, Philadelphia, pp. 1101-1152.

[16] Apte-Sengupta S, Sirohi D, Kuhn RJ (2014) Coupling of replication and assembly in flaviviruses. *Current Opinion Virology* 9:134-142.

[17] Klema VJ, Padmanabhan R, Choi KH (2015) Flaviviral replication complex: coordination between RNA synthesis and 5'-RNA capping. *Viruses* 7: 4640-4656.

[18] Miorin L, Maiuri P, Marcello A (2015) Visual detection of Flavivirus RNA in living cells. *Methods* 98:82-90. http://dx.doi.org/10.1016/j.ymeth.2015.11.002.

[19] Padmanabhan R, Strongin AY (2010) Translation and processing of the dengue virus polyprotein. In: Hanley KA, Weaver SC (Eds.), *Frontiers in Dengue Virus Research*. Caister Academic Press, Norfolk, U.K, pp. 14-33.

[20] Padmanabhan R, Takhampunya R, Teramoto T, Choi KH (2015) Flavivirus RNA synthesis in vitro. *Methods* 91:20-34.

[21] Gupta AK, Kaur K, Rajput A, Dhanda SK, Sehgal M, Khan MS, Monga I, Dar SA, Singh S, Nagpal G, Usmani SS, Thakur A, Kaur G, Sharma S, Bhardwaj A, Qureshi A, Raghava GPS, Kumar M (2016) ZikaVR: An Integrated Zika Virus Resource for Genomics, Proteomics, Phylogenetic and Therapeutic Analysis. *Science Report* 6:32713. doi:10.1038/srep32713.

[22] Devillers J (ed.) (2018) *Computational Design of Chemicals for the Control of Mosquitoes and Their Diseases*, CRC Press, Taylor & Francis Group, Boca Raton, FL, USA.

[23] Bhattacharjee AK (2018) Pharmacophore modeling applied to mosquito-borne diseases. In: Devillers J (Ed), *Computational Design of Chemicals for the Control of Mosquitoes and Their Diseases*, CRC Press, Taylor & Francis Group, Boca Raton, FL, USA, pp. 139-169.

[24] Kapetanovic IM (2008) Computer-aided drug discovery and development (CADDD): in silico-chemico-biological approach. *Chemico-Biological Interactions* 171(2):165-176.

[25] Janseen D (2002) The power of prediction. *Drug Discov*ery 38.

[26] Podlogar BL, Muegge I, Brice LJ (2001) Computational methods to estimate drug development parameters. *Current Opinion Drug Discovery* 12:102-109.

[27] Garcia-Domenech R, Zanni R, Galvez-Llompart M, Galvez J (2018) Molecular topology as a powerful tool for searching for new repellents and novel drugs against diseases transmitted by mosquitoes. In: Devillers J (Ed), *Computational Design of Chemicals for the Control of Mosquitoes and Their Diseases*, CRC Press, Taylor & Francis Group, Boca Raton, FL, USA, pp. 107-137.

[28] (a) Paul SM, Mytelka DS, Dunwiddie CT, Persinger CC, Munos BH, Lindborg SR, Schacht AL (2010) How to improve R&D productivity: the pharmaceutical industry's grand challenge. *Nature Reviews Drug Discovery* 9(3):203-214; (b) Kubinyi H (2006) Success stories of computer-aided design, in Computer Applications. In: Ekins S, Wang B (Eds.) *Pharmaceutical Research and Development*, Wiley-Interscience, pp. 377-424.

[29] Dror O, Shulman-Peleg A, Nussinov R, Wolfso HJ (2004) Predicting molecular interactions in silico: I. A guide to pharmacophore identification and its applications to drug design. *Current Medicinal Chemistry* 11:71-90.

[30] Ehrlich E (1909) Über den jetzigen Stand der Chemotherapie. [About the current state of chemotherapy] *Berichte der deutschen chemischen Gesellschaft* 42(1):17 – 47.

[31] (a) Kier LB (1967) Molecular orbital calculation of preferred conformations of acetylcholine, muscarine, and muscarone. *Molecular Pharmacology* 3(5): 487-494. (b) Gund P (1977) Three dimensional pharmacophore pattern searching. *Progress in Molecular Subcellular Biology* 5:117-143.

[32] Leach AR, Gillet VJ, Lewis RA, Taylor R (2010) Three-Dimensional Pharmacophore Methods in Drug Discovery. *Journal of Medicinal Chemistry* 53:539-558.

[33] Güner OF (Ed.) (2000) *Pharmacophore, perception, development, and use in drug design.* University International Line (IUL Biotechnology Series, San Diego.

[34] Bhattacharjee AK, Hartell MG, Nichols DA, Hicks RP, Stanton B, van Hamont JE, Milhous WK (2004) Structure-activity relationship study of antimalarial indolo [2,1-b]quinazoline-6,12-diones (tryptanthrins). Three dimensional pharmacophore modeling and identification of new antimalarial candidates. *European Journal of Medicinal Chemistry* 39:59-67.

[35] Bhattacharjee AK, Geyer JA, Woodard CL, Kathcart AK, Nichols DA, Prigge ST, Li Z, Mott BT, Waters NC (2004) A three dimensional *in silico* pharmacophore model for inhibition of *plasmodium falciparum* cyclin dependent kinases and discovery of different classes of novel pfmrk specific inhibitors. *Journal of Medicinal Chemistry* 47:5418-5426.

[36] Bhattacharjee AK (2007) Virtual screening of compound libraries using *in silico* three dimensional pharmacophores to aid the discovery and design of antimalarial and antileishmanial Agents. *Frontiers in Drug Design and Discovery* 3:257-292.

[37] Bhattacharjee AK, Marek E, Le HT, Gordon RK (2012) Discovery of non-oxime reactivators using an *in silico* pharmacophore model of oxime reactivators of OP-inhibited acetylcholinesterase. *European Journal of Medicinal Chemistry* 49:229-238.

[38] Buchwald P, Bodor N (2002) Computer-aided drug design: the role of quantitative structure-property, structure-activity and structure-metabolism relationships (QSPR, QSAR, QSMR). *Drug Future* 27:577-588.

[39] Kumar G, Banerjee T, Kapoor N, Surolia N, Surolia A (2010) SAR and Pharmacophore Models for the Rhodanine Inhibitors of Plasmodium falciparum Enoyl-Acyl Carrier Protein Reductase. *Life* 62:204–213.

[40] [Brust A, Palant E, Croker DE, Colless B, Drinkwater R, Patterson B, Schroeder CI, Wilson D, Nielson CK, Smith MT, Alewood D, Alewood PF, Lewis RJ (2009) γ-Conopeptide pharmacophore development: toward a novel class of norepinephrin transporter inhibitor (Xen2174) for pain. *Journal Medicinal Chemistry* 52:6991–7002.

[41] Ren JX, Li LL, Zou J, Yang L, Yang JL, Yang SY (2009) Pharmacophore modeling and virtual screening for the discovery of new transforming growth factor b type I receptor (ALK5) inhibitors. *European Journal of Medicinal Chemistry* 44:4259–4265.

[42] Chen JJ, Liu TL, Yang LJ, Li LL, Wei YQ, Yang SY (2009) Pharmacophore modeling and virtual screening studies of Checkpoint kinase 1 inhibitors. *Chemical and Pharmaceutical Bulletin* 57:704–709.

[43] Ariens EJ (1966) Molecular pharmacology, a basis for drug design. *Progress in Drug Research* 10:429.

[44] Wolber G, Seidel T, Bendix F, Langer T (2008) Molecule-pharmacophore superpositioning and pattern matching in computational drug design. *Drug Discovery Today* 13:23-29.

[45] Walters WP, Stahl MT, Murko MA (1998) Virtual screening - an overview. *Drug Discovery Today* 3:160-178.

[46] Lyne PD (2002) Structure-based virtual screening - a review. *Drug Discovery Today* 7:1047-1055.

[47] Temml V, Kaserer T, Kutil Z, Landa P, Vanek T, Schuster D (2014) Pharmacophore modeling for COX-1 and -2 inhibitors with LigandScout in comparison to Discovery Studio. *Future Medicinal Chemistry* 6:1869-1881.

[48] Discovery Studio (2007) DS Version 2.5, *Accelrys Inc.*, San Diego, CA. http://accelrys.com/products/discovery-studio/.

[49] CATALYST (2000) version 4.10, *Accelrys Inc.*, San Diego, CA. http://www.accelrys.com.

[50] Bhattacharjee AK, Marek E, Le HT, Ratcliffe R, DeMar JC, Pervitsky D, Gordon RK (2015) Discovery of non-oxime reactivators using an in silico pharmacophore model of oxime reactivators of OP-inhibited acetylcholinesterase. *European Journal of Medicinal Chemistry* 90:209-220.

[51] Bhattacharjee AK (2014) Role of in silico stereoelectronic properties and pharmacophores in aid of discovery of novel antimalarials, antileishmanials, and insect Repellents. In: Basak SC, Restrepo G, Villaveces JL (E-book) (Eds), *Advances in Mathematical Chemistry*

and Applications, Bentham Science Publishers, Amsterdam 1:273-305.

[52] Balasubramanian A, Teramoto T, Kulkarni AA, Bhattacharjee AK, Padmanabhan R (2017) Antiviral activities of selected antimalarials against dengue virus type and Zika virus. *Antiviral Research* 137:141-150. (b) Structure of zika virus (5 April 2016) Virology blog, about viruses and viral diseases.

[53] Delvecchio R, Higa LM, Pezzuto P, Valadao AL, Garcez PP, Monteiro FL, Loiola EC, Dias AA, Silva FJM, Aliota MT, Caine EA, Osorio JE, Bellio M, O'Connor DH, Rehen S, de Aquiar RS, Savarino A, Campanati L, A. Tanuri A (2016) Chloroquine inhibits Zika virus infection in different cellular models. *Virus* 8:E322.

[54] Barbosa-Lima G, da Silveira Pinto LS, Kaisar CR, Wardell JL, De Freitas CS, Vieira YR, Marttorelli A, Neto JC, Bozza PT, Wardell SMSV, de Souza MVN, Souza TML (2017) N-(2-arylmethylimino) ethyl-7-chloroquinolin-4-amine derivatives, synthesized by thermal and ultrasonic means, are endowed with anti-Zika virus activity. *European Journal of Medicinal Chemistry* 127:434-441.

[55] Bhattacharjee AK, Kyle DE, Vennerstrom JL, Milhous WK (2002) A 3D QSAR pharmacophore model and quantum chemical structure activity analysis of chloroquine(CQ)-resistance reversal. *Journal of Chemical Information and Computational Science* 42:1212-1220.

[56] Bhattacharjee AK, Kyle DE, Vennerstrom JL (2001) Structural Analysis of Chloroquine-Resistance Reversal by Imipramine Analogs. *Antimicrobial Agents and Chemotherapy* 45:2655-2657.

[57] Vippagunta, SR, Dorn A, Matile H, Bhattacharjee AK, Karle JM, Ellis WY, Ridley RG, Vennerstrom JL (1999) Structural Specificity of Chloroquine-Hematin Binding Related to Inhibition of Hematin Polymerization and Parasite Growth. *Journal of Medicinal Chemistry* 42:4630-4639.

[58] O'Neill PM, Barton VE, Ward SA, Chadwick J (2012) 4-aminoquinolines: chloroquine, amodiaquine and next-generation analogues. In: Staines HM, Krishna S (Eds.), *Treatment and*

Prevention of Malaria. Springer Basel AG. http://dx.doi.org/10.1007/978-3-0346-0480-2_2.

[59] O'Neill PM, Mukhtar A, Stocks PA, Randle LE, Hindley S, Ward SA, Storr RC, Bickley JF, O'Neil IA, Maggs JL, Hughes RH, Winstanley PA, Bray PG, Park BK (2003) Isoquine and related amodiaquine analogues: a new generation of improved 4-aminoquinoline antimalarials. *Journal of Medicinal Chemistry* 46:4933-4945.

[60] O'Neill PM, Park BK, Shone AE, Maggs JL, Roberts P, Stocks PA, Biagini GA, Bray PG, Gibbons P, Berry N, Winstanley PA, Mukhtar A, Bonar-Law R, Hindley S, Bambal RB, Davis CB, Bates M, Hart TK, Gresham, SL, Lawrence RM, Brigandi RA, Gomez-delas-Heras FM, Gargallo DV, Ward SA (2009) Candidate selection and preclinical evaluation of N-tert-butyl isoquine (GSK369796), an affordable and effective 4-aminoquinoline antimalarial for the 21st century. *Journal of Medicinal Chemistry* 52:1408-1415.

[61] Devillers J (2018) Repurposing of insecticides and drugs for the control of mosquitoes and diseases. In: Devillers J (Ed), *Computational Design of Chemicals for the Control of Mosquitoes and Their Diseases*, pp 16-20, CRC Press, Taylor & Francis Group, Boca Raton, FL, USA.

[62] Pascoalino BS, Courtemanche G, Cordeiro MT, Laura HVG, Lucio Freitas-Junior G *(2016)* Zika antiviral chemotherapy: identification of drugs and promising starting points for drug discovery from an FDA-approved library. *F1000 Research* 5:2523 (doi: 10.12688/f1000research.9648.1).

[63] Saiz J-C, Martín-Acebes M-A (2017) The Race To Find Antivirals for Zika Virus. *Antimicrobial Agents and Chemotherapy* 61:e00411-17. https://doi.org/10.1128/AAC.00411-17.

[64] Gaurav A, Gautam V (2014) Structure-based three-dimensional pharmacophores as an alternative to traditional methodologies. *Journal of Receptor, Ligand and Channel Research* 7: 27-38.

[65] Barba-Spaeth G, Dejnirattisai W, Rouvinski1 A, Vaney MC, Medits I, Sharma A, Simon-Lorière E, Sakuntabhai A, Van-Mai Cao-Lormeau VM, Haouz A, England P, Stiasny K, Mongkolsapaya J, Heinz FX,

Screaton GR, Rey FA (2016) Structural basis of potent Zika–dengue virus antibody cross-neutralization. *Nature* http://dx.doi.org/10.1038/nature18938.

[66] Mottin M, Braga RC, da Silva RA, da Silva JHM, Perryman AL, Ekins S, Andrade CH (2017) Molecular Dynamics simulations of Zika Virus NS3 helicase: Insights into RNA binding site activity. *Biochemical and Biophysical Research Communications* DOI: 10.1016/j.bbrc.

[67] Oguntade S, Ramharack P, Soliman MES (2017) Characterizing the ligand-binding landscape of Zika NS3 helicase-promising lead compounds as potential inhibitors. *Future Virology* 12(6): 261–273.

[68] Hercík K, Kozak J, Sala M, Dejmek M, Hrebabecký H, Zborníkov E, Smola M, Ruzek D, Nencka R, Boura E (2017) Adenosine triphosphate analogs can efficiently inhibit the Zika virus RNA-dependent RNA polymerase. *Antiviral Research* 137:131-133.

[69] Munjal A, Khandia R, Dhama K, Sachan S, Karthik K, Tiwari R, Malik YS, Kumar D, Singh RK, Iqbal HMN, Joshi SK (2017) Advances in developing therapies to combat Zika virus: current knowledge and future perspectives. *Frontiers in Microbiology*, www.frontiersin.org, 8: Article 1469.

[70] Barrows NJ, Campos RK, Powell ST, Prasanth KR, Schott-Lerner G, Soto-Acosta R, Galarza-Munoz G, McGrath EL, Urrabaz-Garza R, Gao J, Wu P, Menon R, Saade G, Fernandez-Salas I, Rossi SL, Vasilakis N, Routh A, Bradrick SS, Garcia-Blanco MA (2016) A Screen of FDA-Approved Drugs for Inhibitors of Zika Virus Infection. *Cell Host & Microbe* 20:259–270.

[71] Ekins S, Mietchen D, Coffee M, Stratton TP, Freundlich JS, Freitas-Junior L, Muratov E, Siqueira-Neto J, Williams AJ, Andrade C (2016) Open drug discovery for the Zika virus. *F1000Research* 5:150.

[72] Micewicz ED, Khachatoorian R, French SW, Ruchala P (2018) Identification of novel small-molecule inhibitors of Zika virus infection. *Bioorganic & Medicinal Chemistry Letters* 28 (3):452-458.

[73] Ncube NB, Ramharack P, Soliman MES (2018) An "All-In-One" Pharmacophoric Architecture for the Discovery of Potential Broad-Spectrum Anti-Flavivirus Drugs. *Applied Biochemistry and*

Biotechnology 185(3)799-814, https://doi.org/10.1007/s12010-017-2690-2).

[74] Saiz J-C, Martín-Acebes MA (2017) The Race To Find Antivirals for Zika Virus. *Antimicrobial Agents and Chemotherapy* 61(6):411-17.

[75] Baronti C, Piorkowski G, Charrel RN, Boubis L, Leparc-Goffart I, de Lamballerie X (2014) Complete coding sequence of zika virus from a French polynesia outbreak in 2013. *Genome Announcement* 2(3):e00500–14.

[76] Upadhyay AK, Cyr M, Longenecker K, Tripathi R, Sun C, Kempf DJ (2017) Crystal structure of full-length Zika virus NS5 protein reveals a conformation similar to Japanese encephalitis virus NS5. *Acta Crystallographica* F73:116–122.

[77] Bhattacharjee AK (2007) *In silico* 3D pharmacophores for aiding discovery of the *Pfmrk* (*Plasmodium* Cyclin-dependent protein kinases) specific inhibitors for therapeutic treatment of malaria. *Expert Opinion on Drug Discovery* 2(8):1115-1127.

[78] Sarukhanyan E, Shityakov S, Dandekar T (2018) In Silico Designed Axl Receptor Blocking Drug Candidates Against Zika Virus InfectionIn Silico Designed Axl Receptor Blocking Drug Candidates Against Zika Virus Infection. *ACS Omega* 3:5281−5290.

In: Zika Virus Surveillance …
Editors: Subhash C. Basak et al.
ISBN: 978-1-53614-970-8

Chapter 3

ZIKA VIRUS: THE QUEST FOR VACCINES

***Proyasha Roy*[1], *Ashesh Nandy*[1,*] *and Subhash C. Basak*[2]**
[1]Centre for Interdisciplinary Research and Education, Kolkata, India
[2]Department of Chemistry and Biochemistry,
University of Minnesota Duluth, Duluth, Minnesota, US

ABSTRACT

The sudden rise of Zika virus infections that grew to a pandemic status in the Americas in 2015-16 took the scientific community and public health authorities by surprise. There were no drugs or vaccines to control the intensity and spread of the disease which caused irreparable harm and numerous fatalities. Although the viral cases have died down, research is going on unabated to develop viable drugs and vaccines. In this chapter, we recount the efforts and progress being made to develop suitable vaccines against the Zika virus. We give a brief account of the classical vaccine strategies of live attenuated, inactivated and VLP vaccines and then discuss, in some detail, the latest results in the promising new approach of peptide vaccinology.

* Corresponding Author E-mail: anandy43@yahoo.com.

Keywords: peptide vaccine, Zika virus, graphical representation, vaccine design protocol, vaccinomics, reverse vaccinology, epitope prediction, peptide vaccine problems, vaccine history, inactivated viruses, live attenuated viruses, subunit vaccines, RNA virus

INTRODUCTION

Protective measures against viral infections take two forms: drug administration post-infection, and vaccines at the pre-infection stage, preparing the body's immune capabilities to combat the infection. No drugs or vaccines have yet been found satisfactory for the Zika viral infections. The previous chapter, Chapter 2 of this book, recounted the drug discovery attempts against the Zika virus (ZIKV). In this chapter we recount the quest for suitable vaccines. We begin with a brief history of vaccine origins, narrate the different kinds of vaccines that are in use, relate the traditional types of vaccines that are being tried against the Zika virus and then discuss in some detail the modern approach of peptide vaccines.

Historical Background

Vaccination, in theory, was recognized as far back as around 400 BCE in Greece by Thucydides who noticed that Greek survivors of smallpox infection did not fall victim to the deadly virus a second time [1]. It took a few more centuries for the Chinese and Indians to understand and make use of variolation or inoculation, which essentially utilized infectious microbes in limited quantity to induce an immune reaction, to treat smallpox. In 900-1000 CE, these ancient civilizations would extract scab tissues from patients infected with smallpox, grind the tissue to powder form and insert it up the noses of healthy people - one of the more popular methods of variolation at that time [2-7]. Mild symptoms would develop although they would subside in a few weeks. From the Far East, variolation travelled to the Middle East before it reached England in the 1700's, championed by Italian physician

Emmanuel Timoni of Constantinople and Lady Mary Wortley Montagu [8]. Although variolation did not provide 100% protection and led to eventual death in many cases, it was able to reduce the incidence of the most morbid infectious disease in the world at that time. By 1768, an English physician, John Fewster had noticed the link between prior cowpox infection and subsequent protection from smallpox [9]. Several other physicians, in England and Germany, tested out these observations and observed successful results [10]. It was scientist and physician, Edward Jenner who was responsible for the methodical inquiry into vaccination which led to the subsequent worldwide awareness [11] and the eventual eradication of smallpox in 1979 by the World Health Organization's massive global Smallpox Eradication Campaign [12]. Louis Pasteur and Emile Roux took Jenner's mantle and discovered the rabies vaccine constructed from live attenuated or weakened living rabies virus extracted from infected rabbits in 1885 [13]. The 19th century further saw vaccines developed against typhoid, cholera and the bubonic plague. The 20th century included vaccine discoveries for polio, mumps, measles, pneumonia, rubella, meningitis, hepatitis B, tick-borne encephalitis, Japanese encephalitis among many more [14]. The 21st century not only gave rise to vaccines against several more diseases like human papillomavirus, rotavirus and zoster but also more effective and improved vaccines for cholera, pneumonia and meningitis.

Types of Vaccines

The term "vaccine" was coined by Edward Jenner from the name for smallpox of the cow (*Variolae vaccinae)* and a method was established for production of vaccines. Over time different forms of vaccines were explored and today there are broadly four types of vaccines, which include live attenuated, inactivated, purified proteins or polysaccharides and genetically engineered vaccines.

Live attenuated vaccine (LAIV) has its roots in variolation. Louis Pasteur and his colleagues laid down the foundation for attenuated organisms to be used as immunity builders against the deadly disease-causing microbes which ultimately led to the discovery of the rabies vaccine [13]. These vaccines contain pathogenically weakened microbes that are still alive. The pathogens are weakened by growing them in a foreign host, which are usually tissue cultures, embryonated eggs or live animals. The pathogen adapts to the new host and due to corresponding mutations, that selectively allowed the microbe to survive in the new biological system, it becomes less pathogenic to its initial original host, therefore, making it safe and functional enough to elicit an immunological reaction in the vaccinated individuals.

In vitro serial dilution through artificial media by Calmette and Guérin produced the first effective and attenuated bacterial strain used to treat tuberculosis [15]. Discovery of viral growth in cell culture greatly accelerated the field of vaccination. This method allowed researchers and scientists to selectively grow mutants with low pathogenicity and high immunogenicity. The vaccine for yellow fever virus, a typical virus of the Flavivirus genus that includes the Zika, Dengue and other viruses, was obtained by serial passage in animal models and tissues [16]. The Japanese encephalitis, also of the Flaviviridae family, vaccine strain SA14-14-2 is another example [17]. Influenza vaccines also have been created by using cold-adapted strains which show loss of virulence with adaptation to growth in low temperatures [18]. The rate of reproduction of these less virulent strains will now be low and slow. Due to this reason, individuals require subsequent vaccinations or booster doses to increase the protective immunity. Other than passage through cell cultures, the strains are also weakened by targeted mutations or deletions. However, there are certain disadvantages to these vaccines like the chance of reversion to virulence which may arise from secondary mutations. Moreover, these vaccines absolutely cannot be administered to individuals whose immune system is deficient or weak, also known as immunocompromised/immunodeficient.

In contrast to attenuated vaccines, inactivated or killed vaccines comprise the whole pathogen whose virulence has been reduced by removing their replication machinery using heat, chemicals, detergents or radiation or subunits of the microbe which contain only purified antigens effective to mount an immune response. These inactivated vaccines are weaker than the live vaccines and must be supplemented by booster shots and adjuvants. Adjuvants may be inorganic aluminum salts or organic oil-based. The polio Salk vaccine is an example of inactivated viral vaccine [19]. The first influenza vaccine consisted of a chemically-inactivated virus. Vaccine for the tick-borne encephalitis disease was an addition to the repertoire of inactivated whole or subunits of virus vaccines. Extreme care is taken to properly inactivate whole pathogens lest it remains highly infectious.

Reassortment is another method which has been employed to manufacture the rotavirus vaccines. RNA segments obtained from a bovine rotavirus and one surface protein encoding gene segment from human rotaviruses led to a pentavalent rotavirus vaccine [20]. These methods allowed for attenuated viruses to remain functional enough to evoke a neutralizing immune reaction once injected into the host. Present day attenuated viral vaccines are largely generated by growing viruses in fertilized chicken eggs. The viruses are then disintegrated with detergents and the proteins are purified which serve as protein-based vaccines (e.g., hemagglutinin-based influenza vaccine) [21]. Genetically engineered vaccines have ushered a new era of vaccinology. The first of its kind was the Hepatitis B vaccine which was produced by inserting the surface protein (S) encoding gene sequence into yeast cells. The cells produced this protein in large quantities which were then extracted and purified. Apart from yeast cells, viruses themselves have been used as vectors which express proteins as vaccine antigens. Immunization against the Japanese encephalitis virus (JEV) is precipitated by an attenuated strain of yellow fever virus, 17D yellow fever strain, acting as the vector for two genes (prM and E) of JEV [22]. The human papillomavirus (HPV) vaccine represents a completely new chapter of vaccinology, in that, it consists of virus-like particles (VLPs) [23]. The VLPs are the L1 proteins of HPV which can assemble among themselves into immunogenic aggregates that are much more potent than the natural protein itself [24].

Challenges of Current Vaccines

The majority of the vaccines are produced by the two pharmaceutical giants Sanofi Pasteur and GlaxoSmithKline. From a business point of view, vaccine production is an agreeable venture because the quest to eradicate diseases has no imminent end in sight - both known and unknown. With new discoveries and research into microbiology and physiology of animals, current vaccines have many opportunities for improvement. The current growing population itself lays out an ever-present demand for vaccines. However, there are certain, if not many, challenges posed by the standard vaccine technology:

1. Maintenance of viability of live weakened vaccine strains throughout the manufacturing and supply process.
2. In case of inactivated vaccines which are grown in cell culture, it is imperative to take care that the strains are completely inactivated as well as maintaining their immunogenic potential.
3. In case of purified proteins, the detoxification (i.e., removal of any contaminant) and consistency of the production must be maintained.
4. Carrier proteins required for polysaccharide conjugates need to be constructed in such a manner so as to avoid any intrusion into the immunological activity.
5. Recombinant proteins increase the chances of host protein contamination.
6. Vaccines which are vector-based constitute the threat of reversion or unprecedented genetic behaviour including rearrangement.

While some vaccine production, like that of polio disease, has been optimized and made cost-effective, certain other vaccines, like multivalent vaccines, require rigorous quality control, more resources and thus, more expensive investment.

Unfortunately, antiviral vaccines have to contend with a generic problem: such vaccines are often effective for a short period. This is because viruses mutate very fast, especially RNA viruses like influenza and Dengue, a closely related virus belonging to the same Flaviviridae family as the Zika virus, which statistically would have at least one base in the RNA genome mutated at every replication cycle. The rate is much lower for DNA viruses which have the error correction mechanism at replication; RNA viruses do not have such capacities and therefore errors accumulate very fast [25]. Vaccines against rotavirus have had a chequered history, failing often due to very rapid changes in the sequences. Thus, whatever drugs and vaccines are developed against viral diseases, the high mutation rate that characterizes viral genomes ensure their rapid obsolescence. This necessitates continuous hunt for new drugs and vaccines, but the quest is more complicated by the fact that new viruses from zoonotic sources (e.g., see [26-30]) or elsewhere, e.g., the Nipah virus [31], are constantly emerging with higher frequency, some of which can lead to attacks on human hosts. And without some certainty of adequate markets, commercial interests will not develop.

Immune Response in Brief

Let us take a moment to understand how vaccines work through an organism's immune system to respond to a viral outbreak. The immunity system of organisms recognizes invading pathogens and inhibits them or develops antibodies to fight against them. Innate immunity is the process where the invading pathogens are inhibited by our skin, the mucous membranes in the mouth and nostrils, the acidic environment of the stomach; the pathogens that may still enter through cuts and bruises can be destroyed by phagocytes, macrophages and dendritic cells, and expelled. The response is irrespective of the type of invading pathogen.

Adaptive immunity is more specific. Pathogens, known as antigens, that pass the innate immunity barrier into the blood serum and cells of the organism will face humoral immune response and cell-based immune response, respectively. Both responses are mediated by two special cell types produced in the bone marrow: B-lymphocytes (B-cell) and T-lymphocytes (T-cell). The B-cells on leaving the bone marrow express antigen-binding receptors, called antibodies, on their cell surface; the T-cells mature in the thymus and on leaving express unique molecules on their surface, called T-cell receptors, which also bind the antigens under certain conditions. The receptors on each cell are made from random rearrangements of the peptides. Each B-cell and each T-cell will have thousands of identical receptors on their surface, but different for each cell. The antibodies are very specific in their binding to the antigen; a change of one amino acid can destroy the binding. On binding to an antigen, the specific B-cell or T-cell will generate thousands of copies that will bind to the antigen and lead to phagocytosis and eventual elimination. The process may take 5-6 days for the initial response; later attacks will generate the immune response within 1 to 2 days [25, 32].

ZIKA VIRUS VACCINES

The severe pandemic of the Zika virus in the Americas in 2014-15 would necessitate a quick response in terms of drugs and vaccine administration, but as of September 2018, no drugs or vaccines have reached marketable status for the treatment of Zika infections (see review [33]). A Zika vaccine should be capable of eliciting an immune response, most traditionally an antibody neutralizing response, in order to intercept infection. One of the factors to contend with is what is known as antibody dependent enhancement (ADE), which unfortunately is still not well understood. It has been seen that in the case of the Dengue virus a second infection leads sometimes to a magnification of the severity of the disease. Apparently, the antibodies that were to destroy the invading pathogen turns instead to a helper role and lead to Dengue Hemorrhagic Fever or Dengue Shock Syndrome, which can be fatal [34]. Since the Dengue is so closely related to the Zika virus, the possibility of ADE in Zika cannot be discounted. Tsunoda et al. (2016) [35] talks at length of the further complications contributed by ADE in infected ZIKV patients. Furthermore, an ideal Zika vaccine will also possess the efficacy to arrest the onset of Guillain-Barré syndrome which so often has been correlated to Zika infections.

Several categories of vaccines against the Zika are currently in the developmental stages [36]. The NLM website, ClinicalTrials.gov [37], lists 20 different studies of Zika virus vaccine candidates at present. Most of these are in Phase I trial stage or studying safety and immunogenicity of purified inactivated Zika virus vaccines. A DNA vaccine, developed at the Vaccine Research Center of the National Institute of Allergy and Infectious Diseases (NIAID), is being tested in Phase 2 clinical trials in areas with potential or affirmed Zika infection through mosquito transmission, viz., Brazil and Peru in South America, Panama, Costa Rica and Mexico in Central America, and Texas, Puerto Rico and other areas of the United States of America [38]. The vaccine showed reliable results in animal models, eliciting a neutralizing antibody response to artificial infection with the Zika virus. The vaccine consists of a small circular plasmid DNA which contains two surface protein coding genes of Zika (E and prM). After the translation and formation of the two viral proteins inside the host cells, the immune system is activated.

A Zika purified inactivated virus, ZPIV, developed at the Walter Reed Army Institute of Research in Maryland, has reached the clinical in-human trial phase [39]. It is being tested in 9 different countries. The vaccine comprises the whole viral structure that is able to induce an immune response but without the power to replicate, or in other words, devoid of causing any infection and disease inside the body. With the aid of NIAID, the initial testing of ZPIV vaccine protected non-human primate models in a safe manner.

Other promising vaccines [40] that are currently under evaluation in the Phase I clinical trials include a live attenuated chimeric vaccine which consists of a Dengue type 4 virus onto which Zika surface protein are being artificially expressed, being developed by NIAID's Laboratory of Viral Diseases and a multi-effective vaccine, termed as AGS-v produced by London based SEEK pharmaceutical company that constitutes four mosquito salivary proteins which will prompt an immune response to infected mosquito bites instead of targeting the pathogens. Additionally, a live attenuated Zika virus vaccine with a 10-nucleotide deletion in the 3' untranslated region (3'-UTR) have been developed by Shan et al. (2017) [41].

However, the in human phase clinical trial is facing a major concern. With the drastic reduction in naturally Zika-infected people, the number of candidates for the trial is too low to generate statistically significant results [42]. There are proposals by various investigators to artificially infect individuals with the Zika virus in order to test the safety, efficacy and dosage of the ZPIV, but this raises several ethical and moral problems. Pharmaceutical giant Sanofi, who were developing the ZPIV, has arrested all progress with the vaccine, although NIAID will be taking the testing forward.

Another challenge faced by scientists and vaccine developers is the lack of an established animal model for Zika virus studies. There are ambiguous results observed in immunocompetent mice, rhesus monkeys, rabbits and guinea pigs as there are no consistent clinical manifestations of the disease in all of them [43-45]. While mouse brains exhibit cellular degeneration and inclusion bodies in the central nervous systems and temporary viremia and fever ensue in rhesus monkeys, the same cannot be said for the other animal candidates [46]. In ideal immunocompetent models, viremia will be established along with generation of ZIKV antibodies. Despite several experiments developing interferon deficient mice models, ZIKV infection studies have shown distinct differences in results between the models, in that, clinical signs are present in either young mice or adult mice but not both [47].

On the other hand, as with many biological applications, living systems which apparently lead to destruction and death have been strategically taken advantage of and put to beneficial use. Viral immunotherapy is one such field of application. ZIKV is known to possess oncolytic tropism. The work by Chen et al. (2018) [48] demonstrated that using a live attenuated ZIKV vaccine to treat Glioblastoma, which results in one of the most dangerous brain tumours, showed a reduction in intracerebral tumor development and selective killing of glioma stem cells (that cause tumour recurrence) along with antiviral immune response and inflammation. Furthermore, intracerebral injection of the vaccine did not result in neurological or behavioural anomalies when tested in mice. Such a viral vaccine may be a potential therapeutic treatment for Glioblastoma.

A NEW PARADIGM - PEPTIDE VACCINES

The difficulties faced in using traditional vaccines, e.g., high cost and time for development, storage and transportation difficulties, allergenic reactions, the same vaccine irrespective of country and community, have led some researchers to abandon the "one size fits all" concept of vaccination and delve deeper into the processes that make vaccines work and propose new vaccine strategies [49, 50]. The advances in bioinformatics, computing resources, genomic data banks and new understandings of immunology and immunoinformatics are making it possible to consider developing products purposed towards country, community and individual needs. This is especially important for hyper-variable viruses like influenza and coronavirus where traditional vaccines are failing to live up to the requirements and as well as viruses that have become endemic in different regions like Dengue [51]. Therefore, a standard vaccine may not be equally effective in all cases. The new paradigm holds promise to care for these issues by allowing for a rational design of vaccines and the science of "reverse vaccinology" [52] oriented towards individual, community and population specificity.

The concept of peptide vaccines arose from these approaches. Consider that an organism's immune system seeks to destroy invading pathogens through B-cell and T-cell mechanisms as explained earlier. These cells will target surface proteins of the virus, more specifically certain regions of the protein, termed as epitopes, which are parts of the amino acid sequence making up the virus particle. The idea is that if we can identify these epitopes of a virus, we can prime the body's immune system by generating specific T-cells and B-cells through exposure to peptides that mimic the epitopes; advances in computer technology and bioinformatics are enablers for this purpose. Since such peptides will be small molecules of 10 to 20 amino acids in length, these peptide vaccines can be manufactured synthetically, assure high standards of purity and integrity while maintaining low costs; problems related to storage and transport can also be averted [53]. Even better, any regional variations in the epitopes of an invading pathogen can be easily accommodated, once identified, by making small changes in the peptide during the production process; the process, ideally, can be taken one step further and changes can be made to cover specific individual needs [54].

While the theory seems to be eminently reasonable, peptide vaccines alone do not seem to be able to evoke the immune response that traditional vaccines, with all their faults, can elicit. The reason perhaps lies in the fact that there could be multiple surface accessible epitopes in the pathogen, all of which would have their effects when a live-attenuated virus or an inactivated virus is used as vaccines. This can be countered by effecting multiple peptide vaccines, but that alone does not help either. What seems to be required are (a) carrier proteins on which the peptides can piggyback and (b) addition of adjuvants that act like catalysts to elicit stronger immune response. These and some other issues that arise in prescribing peptide vaccines as preventives against viral infections are remarked upon later in this chapter.

The first successful peptide vaccine to be reported was the canine parvovirus [55], which was followed by developments in malaria [56] and swine fever vaccines for animals [57]. No peptide vaccines for humans have been licensed as yet, but the interest in the new technique is very high. The US National Institute of Health website ClinicalTrials.gov [37] lists 563 studies at various phase trials for peptide vaccines as of 3rd October 2018, a large percentage of which are against various cancers; Singluff (2011) [58], an early proponent of peptide vaccines against cancers, has expressed hope for a very promising future for such vaccines.

Peptide Vaccine Design Protocol

Determining the peptide vaccine requires choosing the appropriate viral protein, selection of the peptide segments according to the researcher's criteria and ensuring they are surface situated, determine the epitopes that best match the recipient population and cross-check against the possibility of autoimmune threats so as to arrive at a final list of suitable peptides (see Flowchart in Figure 3.1). Then comes the wet-lab experiments to test the efficacy of the predictions and to take care of the logistics such as carrier proteins, adjuvants, storage and transport issues, etc.

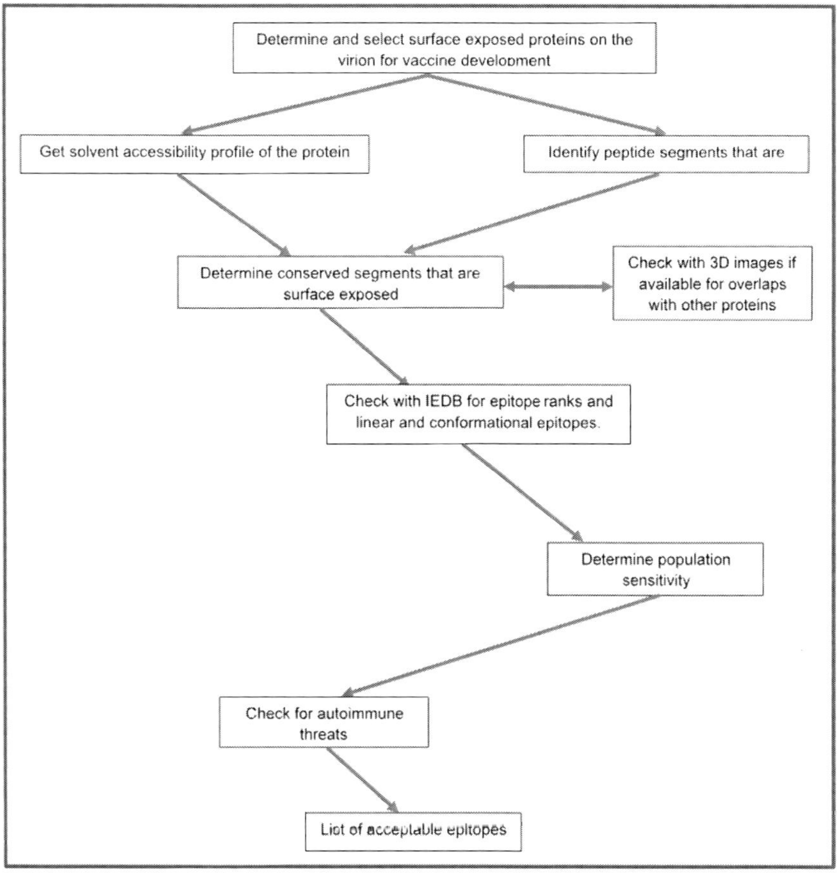

Figure 3.1. Flowchart of peptide vaccine target search protocol.

This procedure has been followed by many to predict and test peptide vaccines for a whole host of viral diseases. Thus, Brossart et al. (2000) [59] showed *in vivo* that a peptide vaccine derived from the human MUC-1 gene encoding cell surface associated mucin benefitted patients with advanced breast and ovarian cancers. Ludewig et al. (2001) [60] found that a peptide vaccine against lymphocytic choriomeningitis virus administered intradermally generated antiviral and antitumor immune response. Liao et al. (2013) [61] demonstrated that epitopes of the human papillomavirus protein E5 predicted by bioinformatics tools, when injected with a suitable adjuvant into mouse muscles, rendered strong cell-mediated immunity and protection from tumor growth. In another mouse model experiment, bioinformatics analysis derived synthetic peptide vaccines showed good protection against Fasciola hepatica virus [62]. A multivalent peptide vaccine consisting of four peptides against non-small cell lung cancer found the vaccine generating strong T-cell response [63].

The search for peptide vaccines against a virus begins with choice of the virion's surface proteins and selection criteria for the peptide segments. The protein sequences are obtained from various databases like NCBI, Virus Variation Resource, UniProt and Virus Pathogen Database and Analysis Resource. The structural proteins are most often the desirable proteins on which predictive analyses are carried out for epitope determination which can then be experimentally verified for antibody response, and thus, induction of host immune response against Zika virus. A necessary step that must be incorporated in the early stages of peptide vaccine design is the identification of conserved regions in the target proteins. Epitopes extracted from immutable regions increases the reliability and stability of the potential vaccine. Traditional routine makes use of multiple sequence alignment (MSA) to find invariable sites conserved across different strains of the virus; ClustalW and Muscle are two of the most popular algorithms used for MSA. For the prediction of epitopes, the Immune Epitope Database (IEDB) [64] hosts a suite of algorithms for predicting B-cell epitopes and T-cell epitopes. B-cell epitopes are characteristically hydrophilic and accessible on the surface for which predictive tools are available in IEDB. Bepipred is a common algorithm for predicting linear B-cell epitopes. The next step is analyzing the binding between the predicted peptide epitope candidates and MHC (Major Histocompatibility Complex) class I and class II molecules. There are various methods by which the binding can be calculated such as Artificial Neural Network, Stabilized Matrix Method, scoring matrices obtained from Combinatorial Peptide Libraries or a combination of all the three represented by the consensus method. A rank-based selection of peptides is made. A complementary step to MHC prediction results is the analysis of the allele coverage of the target population. An ideal coverage would include the majority of the target population or at least the alleles majorly represented in specific target communities.

Using such protocols, Badawi et al. (2016) [65] predicted 3 B-cell epitopes for a potential Zika virus vaccine (amino acid sequences (using one-letter codes) AQDKP, TPNSPRAE and TPHWNNK), 4 MHC class I specific epitopes (MMLELDPPF, MAVLGDTAW, KEWFHDIPL and DTAWDFGSV), 3 MHC class II specific epitopes (FKSLFGGMS, LITANPVIT and VHTALAGAL) and 2 epitopes specific to the South American strains (LDKQSDTQYV and EVQYAGTDGPCK) that are highly recommendable for the development of a therapeutic ZIKV vaccine. Dikhit et al. (2016) [66] identified 63 MHC class I restricted epitopes that bind with 42 HLA supertypes. Based on HLA binding specificity and world-wide population coverage independent of ethnicity, 9 promiscuous epitopes were found with 100% conservation on capsid protein (MVLAILAFL), envelope protein (RLKGVSYSL and RLITANPVI), NS2A (AILAALTPL), NS4B (LLVAHYMYL and LVAHYMYLI) and NS5 (SLINGVVRL, ALNTFTNLV and YLSTQVRYL). Literature review [67-69] has majorly recommended that amino acids 241–259, 294–315, 317–327, 346–361, 377–388 and 421–437 on the envelope protein of ZIKV to be potential peptide vaccine candidates. Similar work has been carried out by Mirza et al. (2016) [68] with envelope, NS3 and NS5 proteins, Shawan et al. (2015) on envelope protein and Dar et al. (2016) [70] with the entire polyprotein of ZIKV.

The disadvantages posed by the peptide vaccines because of the instability of short peptides in serum and low immunogenicity due to rapid degradation post-immunization make it difficult to experimentally test their efficacy. Basu et al. (2018) [71] assessed the potency of the aforementioned highly recommended peptides by expressing them on immunogenic stable bacteriophage virus-like particles or VLPs (MS2, PP7 and Qβ) in mice. The murine host produced anti-ZIKV antibodies against all the epitopes chemically conjugated to the VLPs. However, neutralization was not effective against a high dose of ZIKV and immunizations with VLPs displaying only a single epitope slightly decreased ZIKV infection in mice.

Standard vaccine development eliciting a humoral response in the form of neutralizing antibodies has been hypothesized to cause cross-reactive enhancing antibodies, that is, a previous Dengue infection resulting humoral immunity increases subsequent ZIKV infection more than normal with enhanced viral replication in vitro. However, Dos Santos Franco et al. (2017) [72] designed a flavivirus NS5 protein which induces a cellular immune response against both Dengue and ZIKV, independent of antibodies. 19 epitopes with 100% conservation in ZIKV and Dengue were identified for MHC class I and class II alleles in the Brazilian population with population coverage >50% in major tropical areas of the world.

Cunha-Neto et al. (2017) [73] presented a new method of creating cytotoxic T lymphocyte (CTL) vaccines for ZIKV infection based on a protein structure computer model that has been developed to choose epitopes for CTL attack in viruses demonstrating antigenic drift. A subset of predicted MHC class I ZIKV epitopes (24 in envelope protein and 7 in matrix protein), that matched established Dengue class I epitopes, has been shown to elicit a CD8+ attack. Several ZIKV epitopes on the envelope (QPENLEYRIMLSVHGSQHSG and KCRLKMDKLRLKGVSYSLCT) and matrix (SQKVIYLVMILLIAPAYSIR) proteins exhibiting promiscuous binding to HLA class II molecules that might aid in CTL responses have also been identified.

Weltman (2016) [74] added another layer to epitope selection by factoring in the Shannon entropy along with Bepipred scores of B-cell epitopes. A Shannon entropy score of zero (H = 0.0) corresponds to stable and invariant epitopic regions within potential antigenic ZIKV envelope peptides. Envelope protein sequences used for the study were filtered on the basis of both human host and mosquitoes. Weltman reported that peptide regions at H = 0.0 across both the species is indicative of structural or functional curtailment on mutation, thereby making these amino acid segments conserved and, efficient as peptide vaccine candidates. The analysis predicted 7 peptides (amino acids 53-66, 68-80, 86-96, 102-114, 131-145, 206-218 and 220-233) with epitope activity in envelope protein.

In the race to ZIKV vaccine development, Richner et al. (2017) [73] developed a mRNA based ZIKV vaccine that consists of lipid nanoparticles encasing modified mRNA which encodes the target antigen (ZIKV prM-E) and possesses untranslated regions on either end along with a patented nucleoside modification that decreases triggering of the innate immune system in a random manner. The modified mRNA encoded mutations terminated a cross-reactive epitope (FL) in the second ectodomain of the envelope protein. Immunodeficient mice, and subsequently macaque monkeys, were sufficiently and successfully protected from ZIKV infection by the developing neutralizing antibodies. There was a decrease in the cross-reactive antibodies too. One of the major advantages conferred by this vaccine is its high efficiency with just one dosage which is not usually possible by standard vaccinology. Extending on this, it also makes the contemporary vaccine extremely cost-effective.

Designing the Zika Virus Peptide Vaccine

We now consider the process of rational design of peptide vaccines against the Zika virus in some detail [76]. Determining the peptide segments of a viral protein to be analyzed is a crucial step in the entire process. As recounted above, multiple sequence alignment has been the instrument of choice to select the conserved elements for further epitope analysis. However, multiple sequence alignment is a computer resource hungry process that works best in case of small (<100) number of sequences to be compared. Using more sequences to improve the statistics requires an alignment-free approach, which our lab has been involved in for some time [77]. This started with a 2D graphical representation of the gene sequences [78] for a preliminary indication of conserved regions. In this method a nucleotide sequence is represented on a rectangular grid in which the four bases A, C, G, T are assigned to the four cardinal directions, and a sequence is plotted by taking a step say in the negative x-direction for an A, in the positive y-direction for a C, the positive x-direction for a G and in the negative y-direction for a T. Doing this successively for all the bases in a sequence plots out a curve in the 2D space that is characteristic of the base distribution in the sequence. Inspection of such a plot of the influenza H5N1 neuraminidase gene sequences showed an apparently conserved region of 50 bases at the 3'-end [79, 80]. We used this approach to determine exact matches of Zika virus envelope gene fragments to the few full genes available at the time of our study [69].

To get information on conserved segments of the protein sequence, however, we used an extension of the above model to a 20D rectangular grid where each amino acid was assigned to a particular axis and then proceed to plot the sequence in the abstract space in the same manner as before [81]. We defined the weighted average of coordinate values in each direction to arrive at a weighted centre of mass (c.m.) and a distance measure, p_R, from the origin to the c.m. which is taken as a descriptor of the sequence.

$$\mu_1 = \sum_i x_{1i}/N, \mu_2 = \sum_i x_{2i}/N, \ldots \mu_{20} = \sum_i x_{20i}/N$$
$$p_R = \sqrt{\mu_1^2 + \mu_2^2 + \ldots + \mu_{20}^2}$$

where x_{ji} is the co-ordinate of the jth amino acid, $j = 1, 2, \ldots, 20$, $i = 1, 2, 3, \ldots, N$, N is the length of the protein sequence and p_R is the graph radius from the origin to the centre of mass. While the absolute value of p_R is not material here, it turns out to be very useful in sequence comparison. The p_R, with some computational safeguards, turns out to be characteristic of a sequence and identical sequences will have the same p_R value. We therefore compute the p_R for a short peptide window and then move the window along the sequence to the end to generate a string of p_R values; the size of the window is set at 10 to 14 amino acids in length based on specific HLA parameters. Then we do the same for the next sequence and carry on for all the sequences. Finally, comparing the p_R values at each window position for all the sequences give us a profile of how many different p_R values are there at each position, which implies that the less the variety the more conserved the segment covered by the window. Because of this simple mathematical procedure, it is possible to scan hundreds and thousands of sequences and compare the peptide segments to determine the most conserved peptides. In our research for rational design of peptide vaccines against various viral diseases, we have done this analysis for the H5N1 neuraminidase sequences

[82] where we scanned 514 samples and compared with 425 sequences of H1N1 swine flu neuraminidases. For rotavirus [82] we scanned 438 complete sequences of VP7 surface glycoprotein and for human papillomavirus all available 222 sequences of the L1 capsid gene of various HPV types [83].

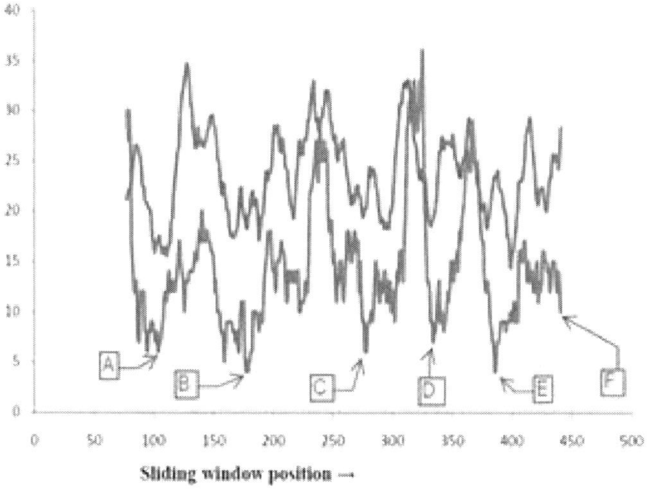

Figure 3.2. A typical chart of ASA profile matching with peptide variability. In this chart analyzing H5N1 neuraminidase proteins, average solvent accessibility (ASA) shown in red is compared with graphical sliding window method (GSWM) generated amino acid segment variability shown in blue. The y-axis represents both the variability and solvent accessibility. The x-axis represents the sliding window middle position number. Reproduced from Ghosh et al. 2010 under CC license.

Comparing a smoothed-out profile of peptide variety variation across the protein sequence with a similarly smoothed out average solvent accessibility (ASA) profile of the protein sequence, we can select the regions where the peptide variety is least (implying most conserved peptide sequence) and the ASA is highest implying greater solvent accessibility. Figure 3.2 shows, for example, a graph displaying this process where we were comparing the ASA and peptide variety profiles for the N1 neuraminidase protein of H5N1 which identified six regions that met our criteria [80]. In the case of our original analysis of the 60 Zika virus envelope proteins where the majority of sequences available were envelope protein fragments [76], we identified four peptide segments that matched our criteria of highly conserved surface exposed segments. The peptides identified by this process are then projected on a 3D structure if available to ensure they are surface accessible; Figure 3.3 shows the six peptides of the H5N1 neuraminidase protein marked on the 3D structure of the protein demonstrating that they are indeed surface situated to a large extent. A similar exercise with the Zika virus 3D structure [84] showed that all the four identified peptide segments had presence on the surface of the protein [76].

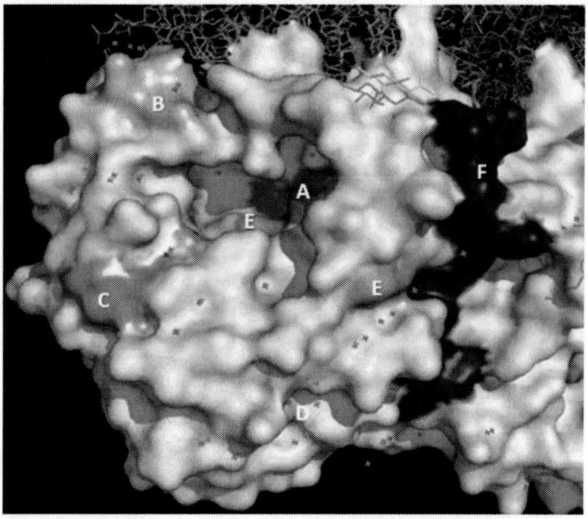

Figure 3.3. Distribution of conserved sequence stretches on neuraminidase surface portions of the highly conserved segments determined from Fig 3.2. Last 16 amino acid corresponding to point F of Fig 3.2 is coloured blue; the amino acid segment corresponding to point A is coloured cherry red, that of point B in pink, point C in dark chocolate, point D in deep salmon and point E in orange. Reproduced (with labels) from Ghosh et al. 2010 under CC license.

The procedures to be followed next depend upon the types and varieties of web-based software available. We used mainly IEDB to determine B-cell and T-cell epitopes based on the HLA allele profile of the target population; of the total results displayed by the IEDB routine, only those that conform to the selected peptides and have low percentile ranks that imply high binding efficiency to the MHC molecules are retained. This procedure generates linear epitopes, but *in vivo* conformational, i.e., discontinuous, epitopes are often the norm. IEDB can also generate conformational epitopes from the given protein sequence; the objective is to ensure that the conformational epitopes also include the peptides identified by the selection process.

The updated list of conserved, solvent accessible peptides with good epitope potential now have to be tested for autoimmune reactions. The standard way is to subject the peptides to a BLAST search to determine if they have any similarities with human proteins, in which case the peptide(s) have to be rejected. The peptides that pass this final test then can be recommended for wet-lab experiments to determine their in vitro and in vivo suitability to evoke the required immune response. For the Zika virus, our analyses [76] identified and recommended four distinct peptides to act as targets for the vaccines: SPRAEATL for the envelope protein amino acid numbers 173 to 180, AGADTGTPHW for aa position 227-236, AAFTFSKVPAE at aa position number 310-320 and MAVDMQTLT at aa 345-353.

In an extension of this exercise, we conducted an analysis of all types of human infecting Flaviviruses, viz., Dengue, Japanese encephalitis, Yellow fever, West Nile virus and the Zika virus, together to determine if a common vaccine can be determined for them [69]. 78 complete envelope protein sequences, including six strains of the Zika virus from recent American epidemic areas, were analyzed through our protocol and four peptide stretches were found in common for the Zika, Dengue and Japanese encephalitis virus. In comparison with the previous exercise for the Zika peptides, the peptides were slightly shifted for the third segment; the other three segments had no parallel since the preliminary study was limited by available fragment extent. Note that the basis for the comparison is not the same: whereas the previous study had African and Asian lineages together, in this case only the Asian-American lineage was used; secondly, this time we were interested in a common vaccine for as many Flaviviruses as we could and therefore the conserved peptide segment and their HLA binding efficiencies were expected to be different. Nevertheless, the peptide segments located in the two studies for the third region are reasonably close.

Our analyses of the influenza neuraminidase genes [80], rotavirus [82], human papillomavirus (HPV) [83] and Zika virus [76] have shown that the surface proteins we have analyzed have yielded four to six peptides that match the criteria we have laid out. Using a large number of sequences in each case to determine the conserved segments implies that peptide vaccines developed on the basis of these segments will remain effective over many cycles of mutations. In the case of the HPV, we were able to recommend sets of peptides that each could cover several types of HPVs. In the case of the Zika virus where two distinct lineages - African and Asian - exist, our original analyses covered all sequences from both lineages available at the time and the peptide segments we determined are common to and conserved in both lineages [76], where generally most researchers concentrate more on one lineage or the other (e.g., see review by Beaver et al. 2018 [85]).

Challenges for Peptide Vaccines

Peptide vaccines are being proposed as alternative to traditional vaccines, being pre-selected for their good epitope potential to elicit immune response. Peptide vaccines being easy to manufacture and cost effective, they can be purified and tailor-made to offset any adverse reactions on a target population, as well as limit any allergenic or reactogenic issues [86]. Peptide vaccines have shown remarkable success in the case of canine parvovirus [55] and have chalked up good success in cancers such as melanoma such that Singluff (2011) [58] remarks that peptide vaccines could be the future cure for cancer.

To date, however, no peptide vaccine has been licensed for use in humans. Such vaccines have been found to have several drawbacks such as (1) need for carriers and adjuvants to stimulate adequate immune response, (2) limitations of single epitope vaccines because of low molecular level of the oligopeptide, (3) lack of efficacy, among others. Cellis (2002) [87] reported that the peptide derived vaccines in certain cases induces "low quality" CTLs (cytotoxic T-lymphocytes) which do not aid killing of diseased cells. There is also the observation that these types of vaccines are used to expose the human body to certain peptides so that its own immunity system will create enough T-cell antibodies to prepare against a subsequent infection. However. a recent study by Liu et al. (2006) [88] on mice have shown that if the body had already been exposed to the original virus, subsequent exposure to the peptide vaccines can create an over-abundant supply of the antibodies. Since T-cells secrete some toxic chemicals, excess of T-cells can be deleterious. In the experiments of Liu et al. (2006) [88], mice exposed to peptide vaccines after initial bout with a virus died. The lesson drawn is that there has to be a recommended dosage to ensure there is no excess of T-cell production.

Doubtless there will be many more challenges this nascent but highly promising approach to rational vaccine design will have to face before it yields superior results and is accepted wholeheartedly. It has the potential to address most infectious and cancerous diseases and with more robust technological and immunological studies this potential can be realized. One can then consider having a string of self-contained peptide vaccine manufacturing labs in susceptible localities where in the case of an epidemic the peptide sequence information can be supplied from a lead lab and which can then manufacture the required vaccine at a fast rate. Also, being designed to cater to local population, the peptide can be primed where possible against endemic pathogens to be more effective for the local population while neighbouring countries can do their own adjustments. With the rapid rise in viral diseases arising from zoonotic and other sources, some such fast response and efficacious capability has to be envisaged for a safe future.

CONCLUSION

The quest for a viable vaccine against the Zika virus is far from over. From repurposing traditional vaccines of viruses [89, 90] from the same Flaviviridae family to new varieties of inactivated vaccines and VLPs, many trials have been and are being conducted. The quiescence of the Zika virus in recent times after the pandemic of 2015-16 is providing a breathing space for development of new vaccines, of which peptide vaccines hold great promise as a harbinger of new trends in antiviral vaccines. The continuous development in computational resources, databases, immunogenetics and related knowledge fields are providing the solid backbone for this research. Yet a lot of ground still has to be covered, a lot of opportunities lie ahead.

Acknowledgments

The authors are grateful to Sumanta Dey and Tathagata Dutta of the Centre for Interdisciplinary Research and Education, Kolkata for providing initial insights and recommendations in the development of this chapter.

References

[1] Henderson, D. A., Moss, B. 1999. "Smallpox and Vaccinia." In *Vaccines,* edited by S. A. Plotkin, W. A. Orenstein, Chapter 6. Philadelphia: Saunders.

[2] Gordon, Charles Alexander. 1884. *An Epitome of the Reports of the Medical Officers to the Chinese Imperial Maritime Customs from 1871 to 1882*. London: Bailliere, Tindall and Cox.

[3] Macgowan DJ. 1884. "Report on the health of Wenchow for the half-year ended 31 March 1884." *China, Imperial Maritime Customs Medical Reports* 27:9–18.

[4] Needham, Joseph. 1980. *China and the origins of immunology.* Centre of Asian Studies. Hong Kong: University of Hong Kong.

[5] Needham, Joseph. 2000. *Science and Civilization in China vol. VI Biology and Biological Technology Part VI Medicine.* Edited by Nathan Sivin. Cambridge: Cambridge University Press.

[6] Boylston, Arthur. 2012. "The origins of inoculation." *Journal of the Royal Society of Medicine* 105(7):309-313.

[7] Lahariya, Chandrakant. 2014. "A brief history of vaccines & vaccination in India." *Indian Journal of Medical Research* 139(4):491–511.

[8] Dinc, Gulten, Ulman, Isil Ulman. 2007. "The introduction of variolation 'A La Turca' to the West by Lady Mary Montagu and Turkey's contribution to this." *Vaccine* 25(21):4261-5.

[9] Thurston, L., Williams, G. 2015. "An examination of John Fewster's role in the discovery of smallpox vaccination." *Journal of the Royal College of Physicians of Edinburgh* 45(2):173-9.

[10] Hammarsten, J. F., Tattersall, W., Hammarsten, J. E. 1979. "Who discovered smallpox vaccination? Edward Jenner or Benjamin Jesty?" *Transactions of American Clinical and Climatological Association* 90:44-55.

[11] Riedel, S. 2005. "Edward Jenner and the History of Smallpox and Vaccination." *Proceedings (Baylor University. Medical Center)* 18(1):21-5.

[12] Fenner, F., Henderson, D. A., Arita, I., Jezek, Z., Ladnyi, I. D. 1988. "*Smallpox and its Eradication*" Geneva: WHO.

[13] Fu, Z. F. 1997. "Rabies and rabies research: past, present and future." *Vaccine* 15:S20-4.

[14] W., Melanie. "*Everything you need to know about vaccines*". Carrington College, California. Accessed September 25, 2018. https://carrington.edu/blog/medical/vaccines/the-20th-century-vaccinations-become-safer-and-many-diseases-vanish/.

[15] Luca, S., Mihaescu, T. 2013. "History of BCG Vaccine." *Mædica* 8(1):53-58.

[16] Frierson, J. G. 2010. "The Yellow Fever Vaccine: A History." *The Yale Journal of Biology and Medicine* 83(2):77-85.

[17] Wiwanitkit, V. 2009. "Development of a vaccine to prevent Japanese encephalitis: a brief review." *International Journal of General Medicine* 2:195-200.

[18] Maassab, H. F., DeBorde, D. C. 1985. "Development and characterization of cold-adapted viruses for use as live virus vaccines." *Vaccine* 3(5):355-69.

[19] Baicus, A. 2012. "History of polio vaccination." *World Journal of Virology* 1(4):108-114.

[20] Clark, H. F., Borian, F. E., Plotkin, S. A. 1990. "Immune protection of infants against rotavirus gastroenteritis by a serotype 1 reassortant of bovine rotavirus WC3." *Journal of Infectious Disease* 161(6):1099-104.

[21] Cate, T. R., Couch, R. B., Kasel, J. A., Six, H. R. 1977. "Clinical trials of monovalent influenza A/New Jersey/76 virus vaccines in adults: reactogenicity, antibody response, and antibody persistence." *Journal of Infectious Disease* 136:S450-5.

[22] Guy, B., Guirakhoo, F., Barban, V., Higgs, S., Monath, T. P., Lang, J. 2010. "Preclinical and clinical development of YFV 17D-based chimeric vaccines against dengue, West Nile and Japanese encephalitis viruses." *Vaccine* 28(3):632-49.

[23] Kirnbauer, R., Booy, F., Cheng, N., Lowy, D. R., Schiller, J. T. 1992. "Papillomavirus L1 major capsid protein elf-assembles into virus-like particles that are highly immunogenic." *Proceedings of National Academy of Sciences of the USA* 89(24):12180-4.

[24] Nascimento, I. P., Leite, L. C. C. 2012. "Recombinant vaccines and the development of new vaccine strategies." *Brazilian Journal of Medical and Biological Research* 45(12): 1102–1111.

[25] Nandy, A., Basak, S. C. 2018. "Bioinformatics in design of antiviral vaccines." *Encyclopedia of Biomedical Engineering - Bioinstrumentation and Bioinformatics,* Elsevier (to be published).

[26] He, B., Fan, Q., Yang, F., Hu, T., Qiu, W., Feng, Y., Li, Z., Li, Y., Zhang, F., Guo, H., Zou, X., Tu, C. 2013. "Hepatitis Virus in Long-Fingered Bats, Myanmar." *Emerging Infectious Disease* 19:638-40.

[27] Kapoor, A., Kumar, A., Simmonds, P., Bhuva, N., Singh, Chauhan L., Lee, B., Sall, A. A., Jin, Z., Morse, S. S., Shaz, B., Burbelo, P .D., Lipkin, W. I. 2015. "Virome Analysis of Transfusion Recipients Reveals a Novel Human Virus That Shares Genomic Features with Hepaciviruses and Pegiviruses." *mBio* 6(5).

[28] Shi, M., Lin, X. D., Tian, J. H., Chen, L. J., Chen, X., Li, C. X., Qin, X. C., Li, J., Cao, J. P., Eden, J. S., Buchmann, J., Wang, W., Xu, J.,

Holmes, E. C., Zhang, Y. Z. 2016. "Redefining the invertebrate RNA virosphere." *Nature* 540:539-543.

[29] Abrahao, J., Silva, L., Silva, L. S., Khalil, J. Y. B., Rodrigues, R., Arantes, T., Assis, F., Boratto, P., Andrade, M., Kroon, E. G., Ribeiro, B., Bergier, I., Seligmann, H., Ghigo, E., Colson, P., Levasseur, A., Kroemer, G., Raoult, D., La Scola, B. 2018. "Tailed giant Tupanvirus possesses the most complete translational apparatus of the known virosphere". *Nature Communications* 9:479.

[30] Kauffman, K. M., Hussain, F. A., Yang, J., Arevalo, P., Brown, J. M., Chang, W. K., VanInsberghe, D., Elsherbini, J., Sharma, R. S., Cutler, M. B., Kelly, L., Polz, M. F. 2018. "A major lineage of non-tailed dsDNA viruses as unrecognized killers of marine bacteria." *Nature* 554:118-122.

[31] Roy, P., Nandy, A. 2018. Nipah Virus–An Epidemic in the Making and a Vaccine Strategy. *Journal of Bacteriology and Vaccine Research* 1(1):1004.

[32] Goldsby, R. A., Kindt, T. J., Osborne, B. A., Kuby, J. 2003. *Immunology* (4th edn.). New York: W H Freeman & Co.

[33] Poland, G. A., Kennedy, R. B., Ovsyannikova, I. G., Palacios, R., Ho, P. L., Kalil, J. 2018. "Development of vaccines against Zika virus." *The Lancet Infectious Diseases* 18:211-219.

[34] Kularatne Senanayake, A. M. 2015. "Dengue fever." *BMJ* 351:h4661.

[35] Tsunoda, I., Omura, S., Sato, F., Kusunoki, S., Fujita, M., Park, A. M., Hasanovic, F., Yanagihara, R., Nagata, S. 2016. "Neuropathogenesis of Zika Virus Infection: Potential Roles of Antibody-Mediated Pathology." *Acta Medica Kinki University* 41(2):37-52.

[36] NIAID. 2018. "Zika virus vaccines". *NIAID*. Accessed August 16, 2018. https://www.niaid.nih.gov/diseases-conditions/zika-vaccines.

[37] ClinicalTrials.gov. 2018. "Peptide vaccines". *ClinicalTrials.gov*. Accessed September 30, 2018. https://clinicaltrials.gov/ct2/results?term=peptide+vaccines &pg=2.

[38] NIAID. 2017. "Phase 2 Zika Vaccine Trial Begins in U.S., Central and South America". *NIAID*. Accessed September 30, 2018. https://www.

niaid.nih.gov/news-events/phase-2-zika-vaccine-trial-begins-us-central-and-south-america.

[39] Modjarrad, K., Lin, L., George, S. L., Stephenson, K. E., Eckels, K. H., De La Barrera, R. A., Jarman, R. G., Sondergaard, E., Tennant, J., Ansel, J. L., Mills, K., Koren, M., Robb, M. L., Barrett, J., Thompson, J., Kosel, A. E., Dawson, P., Hale, A., Tan, C. S., Walsh, S. R., Meyer, K. E., Brien, J., Crowell, T. A., Blazevic, A., Mosby, K., Larocca, R. A., Abbink, P., Boyd, M., Bricault, C. A., Seaman, M. S., Basil, A., Walsh, M., Tonwe, V., Hoft, D. F., Thomas, S. J., Barouch, D. H., Michael, N. L. 2018. "Preliminary aggregate safety and immunogenicity results from three trials of a purified inactivated Zika virus vaccine candidate: phase 1, randomised, double-blind, placebo-controlled clinical trials." *The Lancet* 391:563-571.

[40] Owens, B. 2018. "Zika vaccine development: two years on from the outbreak." *The Pharmaceutical Journal* 300(7910).

[41] Shan, C., Muruato, A. E., Nunes, B. T. D., Luo, H., Xie, X., Medeiros, D. B. A., Wakamiya, M., Tesh, R.B., Barrett, A. D., Wang, T., Weaver, S. C., Vasconcelos, P. F. C., Rossi, S. L., Shi, P. Y. 2017. "A live-attenuated Zika virus vaccine candidate induces sterilizing immunity in mouse models." *Nature Medicine* 23(6):763-767.

[42] Cohen, Joy. 2018. "As massive Zika vaccine trial struggles, researchers revive plan to intentionally infect humans." *Science,* September 2018. Accessed October 2, 2018. https://www.sciencemag.org/news/2018/09/massive-zika-vaccine-trial-struggles-researchers-revive-plan-intentionally-infect.

[43] Dudley, D. M., Aliota, M. T., Mohr, E. L., Weiler, A. M., Lehrer-Brey, G., Weisgrau, K. L., Mohns, M. S., Breitbach, M. E., Rasheed, M. N., Newman, C. M., Gellerup, D. D., Moncla, L. H., Post, J., Schultz-Darken, N., Schotzko, M. L., Hayes, J. M., Eudailey, J. A., Moody, M. A., Permar, S. R., O'Connor, S. L., Rakasz, E. G., Simmons, H. A., Capuano, S., Golos, T. G., Osorio, J. E., Friedrich, T. C., O'Connor, D.H. 2016. "A rhesus macaque model of Asian-lineage Zika virus infection." *Nature Communications* 7(12204).

[44] Dowall, S. D., Graham, V. A., Rayner, E., Atkinson, B., Hall, G., Watson, R. J., Bosworth, A., Bonney, L. C., Kitchen, S., Hewson, R. 2016. "A susceptible mouse model for Zika virus infection." *PLoS Neglected Tropical Diseases* 10(0004658).

[45] Lazear, H. M., Govero, J., Smith, A. M., Platt, D. J., Fernandez, E., Miner, J. J., Diamond, M. S. 2016. "A mouse model of Zika virus pathogenesis." *Cell Host Microbe* 19:720–730.

[46] Dawes, B. E., Smalley, C. A., Tiner, B. L., Beasley, D. W., Milligan, G. N., Reece, L. M., Hombach, J., Barrett, A.D. 2016. "Research and development of Zika virus vaccines." *NPJ Vaccines* 1:16007.

[47] Rossi, S. L., Tesh, R. B., Azar, S. R., Muruato, A. E., Hanley, K. A., Auguste, A.J., Langsjoen, R. M., Paessler, S., Vasilakis, N., Weaver, S. C. 2016. "Characterization of a novel murine model to study Zika virus." *American Journal of Tropical Medicine and Hygiene* 94:1362–1369.

[48] Chen, Q., Wu, J., Ye, Q., Ma, F., Zhu, Q., Wu, Y., Shan, C., Xie, X., Li, D., Zhan, X., Li, C., Li, X. F., Qin, X., Zhao, T., Wu, H., Shi, P. Y., Man, J., Qin, C. F. 2018. "Treatment of Human Glioblastoma with a Live Attenuated Zika Virus Vaccine Candidate." *Mbio* 9(5): e01683-18.

[49] Poland, G. A., Kennedy, R. B., Ovsyannikova, I. G. 2011. "Vaccinomics and personalized vaccinology: Is science leading us toward a new path of directed vaccine development and discovery?" *PLoS Pathogens* 7:e1002344.

[50] Poland, G. A., Whitaker, J. A., Poland, C. M., Ovsyannikova, I. G., Kennedy, R. B. 2016. "Vaccinology in the third millennium: Scientific and social challenges." *Current Opinion in Virology* 17:116–125.

[51] Roy, P., Dey, S., Nandy, A., Basak, S. C., Das, S. 2018. "Base Distribution in Dengue Nucleotide Sequences Differs Significantly from Other Mosquito-Borne Human-Infecting Flavivirus Members." *Current Computer-Aided Drug Design* (ePub ahead of print). doi: 10.2174/1573409914666180731090005.

[52] Rappuoli, R. 2001. "Reverse vaccinology, a genome-based approach to vaccine development. *Vaccine* 19:2688–2691.

[53] Moisa, A. A., Kolesanova, E. F. 2012. "*Synthetic peptide vaccines. An Insight and Control of Infectious Disease in Global Scenario*." Edited by P. Roy. Croatia: InTech.

[54] Nandy, A., Basak, S. C. 2016. "A brief review of computer-assisted approaches to rational design of peptide vaccines." *International Journal of Molecular Sciences* 17(666).

[55] Langeveld, J. P. M., Casal, J. I., Osterhaus, A. D. M. E., Cortés, E., de Swart, R., Vela, C., Dalsgaard, K., Puijk, W.C., Schaaper, W., Meloen, R. H. 1994. "First peptide vaccine providing protection against viral infection in the target animal: Studies of canine parvovirus in dogs." *Journal of Virology* 68:4506-13.

[56] Wang, R., Charoenvit, Y., Corradin, G., Porrozzi, R., Hunter, R. L., Glenn, G., Alving, C. R., Church, P., Hoffman, S. L. 1995. "Induction of protective polyclonal antibodies by immunization with a Plasmodium yoelii circumsporozoite protein multiple antigen peptide vaccine." *Journal of Immunology* 154:2764–2793.

[57] Monso, M., Tarradas, J., de la Torre, B. G., Sobrino, F., Ganges, L., Andreu, D. 2011. "Peptide vaccine candidates against classical swine fever virus: T cell and neutralizing antibody responses of dendrimers displaying E2 and NS2–3 epitopes." *Journal of Peptide Science* 17:24–31.

[58] Singluff, C. L. 2011. "The present and future of peptide vaccines for cancer: Single or multiple, long or short, alone or in combination?" *Cancer Journal* 17:343–350.

[59] Brossart, P., Wirths, S., Stuhler, G., Reichardt, V. L., Kanz, L., Brugger, W. 2000. "Induction of cytotoxic T-lymphocyte responses in vivo after vaccinations with peptide-pulsed dendritic cells." *Blood* 96: 3102–3108.

[60] Ludewig, B., Barchiesi, F., Pericin, M., Zinkernagel, R. M., Hengartner, H., Schwendener, R. A. 2001. "In vivo antigen loading and activation of dendritic cells via a liposomal peptide vaccine mediates protective antiviral and anti-tumour immunity." *Vaccine* 19:23–32.

[61] Liao, S.-J., Deng, D.-R., Zeng, D., Ma, D. 2013. "HPV16 E5 peptide vaccine in treatment of cervical cancer in vitro and in vivo." *Journal of Huazhong University of Science and Technology* 33: 735–742.

[62] Rojas-Caraballo, J., López-Abán, J., Pérez del Villar, L., Vizcaíno, C., Vicente, B., Fernández-Soto, P., del Olmo, E., Patarroyo, M.A., Muro, A. 2014. "*In vitro* and *in vivo* studies for assessing the immune response and protection-inducing ability conferred by fasciola hepatica-derived synthetic peptides containing B- and T-cell epitopes." *PLoS ONE* 9(e105323).

[63] Suzuki, H., Fukuhara, M., Yamaura, T., Mutoh, S., Okabe, N., Yaginuma, H., Hasegawa, T., Yonechi, A., Osugi, J., Hoshino, M., Kimura, T., Higuchi, M., Shio, Y., Ise, K., Takeda, K., Gotoh, M. 2013. "Multiple therapeutic peptide vaccines consisting of combined novel cancer testis antigens and anti-angiogenic peptides for patients with non-small cell lung cancer." *Journal of Translational Medicine* 11(97).

[64] *IEDB Analysis Resource*. http://tools.immuneepitope.org/bcell/.

[65] Badawi, M. M., Osman, M. M., Alla, A. A. E. F., Ahmedani, A. M., Abdalla, M. H., Gasemelseed, M. M., Elsayed, A. A., Salih, M. A. 2016. "Highly Conserved Epitopes of ZIKA Envelope Glycoprotein May Act as a Novel Peptide Vaccine with High Coverage: Immunoinformatics Approach." *American Journal of Biomedical Research* 4(3): 46-60.

[66] Dikhit, M. R., Ansari, M. Y., Vijaymahantesh, K., Mansuri, R., Sahoo, B. R., Dehury, B., Amit, A., Topno, R. K., Sahoo, G. C., Ali, V., Bimal, S., Das, P. 2016. "Computational prediction and analysis of potential antigenic CTL epitopes in Zika virus: A first step towards vaccine development." *Infection, Genetics and Evolution* 45:187-197.

[67] Shawan, M. M. A. K., Mahmud, H. A., Hasan, M. M., Parvin, A., Rahman, M. N., Rahman, S. M. B. 2014. "In Silico Modeling and Immunoinformatics Probing Disclose the Epitope Based Peptide Vaccine Against Zika Virus Envelope Glycoprotein." *Indian Journal of Pharmaceutical and Biological Research* 2(4):44-57.

[68] Mirza, M. U., Rafique, S., Ali, A., Munir, M., Ikram, N., Manan, A., Salo-Ahen, O. M., Idrees, M. 2016. "Towards peptide vaccines against Zika virus: immunoinformatics combined with molecular dynamics simulations to predict antigenic epitopes of Zika viral proteins." *Scientific Reports* 6:37313.

[69] Dey, S., Das, S., Nandy, A. 2017. "Characterization of Zika and Other Human Infecting Flavivirus Envelope Proteins and Determination of Common Conserved Epitope Regions." *EC Microbiology* 8.1: 29-46.

[70] Dar, H., Zaheer, T., Rehman, M. T., Ali, A., Javed, A., Khan, G. A., Babar, M. M., Waheed, Y. 2016. "Prediction of promiscuous T-cell epitopes in the Zika virus polyprotein: An in silico approach." *Asian Pacific Journal of Tropical Medicine* 9(9):844-850.

[71] Basu, R., Zhai, L., Contreras, A., Tumban, E. 2018. "Immunization with phage virus-like particles displaying Zika virus potential B-cell epitopes neutralizes Zika virus infection of monkey kidney cells." *Vaccine* 36(10):1256-1264.

[72] Dos Santos Franco, L., Oliveira Vidal, P., Amorim, J. H. 2017. "In silico design of a Zika virus non-structural protein 5 aiming vaccine protection against zika and dengue in different human populations." *Journal of Biomedical Science* 24:88.

[73] Cunha-Neto, E., Rosa, D. S., Harris, P. E., Olson, T., Morrow, A., Ciotlos, S., Herst, C. V., Rubsamen, R. M. 2017. "An Approach for a Synthetic CTL Vaccine Design against Zika Flavivirus Using Class I and Class II Epitopes Identified by Computer Modeling." *Frontiers in Immunology* 8:640.

[74] Weltman, J. K. 2016. "Computer-Assisted Vaccine Design by Analysis of Zika Virus E Proteins Obtained either from Humans or from Aedes Mosquitos. *Journal of Medical Microbiology and Diagnosis* 5:235.

[75] Richner, J. M., Himansu, S., Dowd, K. A., Butler, S. L., Salazar, V., Fox, J. M., Julander, J. G., Tang, W. W., Shresta, S., Pierson, T. C., Ciaramella, G., Diamond, M. S. 2017. "Modified mRNA vaccines protect against Zika virus infection." *Cell* 168(6):1114-1125.

[76] Dey, S., Nandy, A., Basak, S.C., Nandy, P., Das, S. 2017. "A Bioinformatics approach to designing a Zika virus vaccine." *Computational Biology and Chemistry* 68: 143-152.

[77] Nandy, A. 2014. "The GRANCH Techniques for Analysis of DNA, RNA and Protein Sequences. Advances in Mathematical Chemistry and Applications." Vol. 2, edited by S. C. Basak, G. Restrepo and J. L. Villaveces, 66-94. Bentham Science Publications.

[78] Nandy, A. 1994. "A new graphical representation and analysis of DNA sequence structure: I. Methodology and Application to Globin Genes." *Current Science* 66(4):309-314.

[79] Nandy, A., Basak, S. C. 2010. "New Approaches to Drug-DNA Interactions Based on Graphical Representation and Numerical Characterization of DNA Sequences." *Current Computer-Aided Drug Design* 6:283-289.

[80] Ghosh, A., Nandy, A., Nandy, P. 2010. "Computational analysis and determination of a highly conserved surface exposed segment in H5N1 avian flu and H1N1 swine flu neuraminidase." *BMC Structural Biology* 10:6.

[81] Nandy, A., Ghosh, A., Nandy, P. 2009. "Numerical characterization of protein sequences and application to voltage-gated sodium channel alpha subunit phylogeny." *In Silico Biology* 9:77-87.

[82] Ghosh, A., Chattopadhyay, S., Chawla-Sarkar, M., Nandy, P., Nandy, A. 2012. "In Silico Study of Rotavirus VP7 Surface Accessible Conserved Regions for Antiviral Drug/Vaccine Design." *PLoS ONE* 7(7): e40749.

[83] Dey, S., De, A., Nandy, A. 2016. "Rational Design of Peptide Vaccines Against Multiple Types of Human Papillomavirus." *Cancer Informatics* 15(S1):1–16.

[84] Sirohi, D., Chen, Z., Sun, L., Klose, T., Pierson, T. C., Rossmann, M. G., Kuhn, R. J. 2016. "The 3.8 Å resolution cryo-EM structure of Zika virus." *Science* 352(6284):467-70.

[85] Beaver, J. T., Lelutiu, N., Habib, R., Skountzou, I. 2018. "Evolution of Two Major Zika Virus Lineages: Implications for Pathology,

Immune Response, and Vaccine Development." *Frontiers in Immunology* 9:1640.

[86] Purcell, A. W., McCluskey, J., Rossjohn, J. 2007. "More than one reason to rethink the use of peptides in vaccine design." *Nature Reviews* 6:404–414.

[87] Cellis, E. 2002. "Getting peptide vaccines to work: just a matter of quality control?" *The Journal of Clinical Investigation* 110(12):1765-1768.

[88] Liu, F., Feuer, R., Hassett, D. E., Whitton, J. L. 2006. "Peptide vaccination of mice immune to LCMV or vaccinia virus causes serious CD8+ T cell mediated, TNF-dependent immunopathology." *Journal of Clinical Investigation* 116(2):465-475.

[89] Law, G. L., Tisoncik-Go, J., Korth, M. J., Katze, M. G. 2013. "Drug repurposing: a better approach for infectious disease drug discovery?" *Current Opinion in Immunology* 25(5):588-592.

[90] Rose, M. L., Fehling, C. K. 2017. "How to speed up drug and vaccine development during a public health crisis." *STAT*, November 2017. Accessed 17th October 2018. https://www.statnews.com/2017/11/09/drug-vaccine-development-public-health/.

BIOGRAPHICAL SKETCH

Proyasha Roy

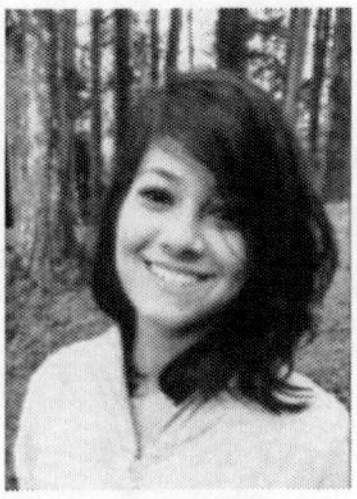

Proyasha Roy completed her Masters in Biotechnology from Bangalore University in 2016. After spending some time at the Indian Institute of

Science, she joined the Centre for Interdisciplinary Research and Education in Kolkata as a Research Intern. With Dr. Ashesh Nandy as mentor, she has worked on analysis of multiple viral genomes using graphical representation and numerical characterization to understand the composition and distribution of bases in nucleic acids and amino acids in proteins. Proyasha has a keen interest specifically in emerging viral diseases and neglected diseases in general.

Publications from the Last 3 Years:

1. Dey, S.; Roy, P.; Nandy, A.; Basak, S.C.; Das, S. (2017). "Comparison of Base Distribution in Dengue, Zika and Other Flavivirus Envelope and NS5 Genes." *MOL2NET 2017*, International Conference on Multidisciplinary Sciences, 3rd edition, 4966. DOI:10.3390/mol2net-03-04966.
2. Roy, P.; Dey, S.; Nandy, A.; Basak, S.C. (2018). "Base Distribution in Dengue Nucleotide Sequences Differs Significantly from Other Mosquito-Borne Human-Infecting Flavivirus Members." *Current Computer-Aided Drug Design*. DOI: 10.2174/ 1573409914666180731090005. (Epub ahead of print).
3. Nandy, A.; De, A.; Roy, P.; Dutta, M.; Roy, M.; Sen, D.; Basak, S.C. (2018). "Alignment-Free Analyses of Nucleic Acid Sequences Using Graphical Representation (with Special Reference to Pandemic Bird Flu and Swine Flu): Omics Tools and Their Applications." In *Synthetic Biology*, edited by Shailza Singh, 141-188. Singapore: Springer.
4. Sen, D.; Roy, P.; Nandy, A.; Basak, S.C.; Das, S. (2018). "Graphical representation methods: How well do they discriminate between homologous gene sequences?" *Chemical Physics* 513:156-164. DOI: https://doi.org/10.1016/j.chemphys.2018.07.031.
5. Nandy, A.; Roy, P. (2018). "Nipah Virus-An Epidemic in the Making and a Vaccine Strategy." *Journal of Bacteriology and Vaccine Research* 1(1):1004.

In: Zika Virus Surveillance …
Editors: Subhash C. Basak et al.
ISBN: 978-1-53614-970-8

Chapter 4

QUANTITATIVE NUCLEIC ACID SEQUENCE COMPARISON METHODS IN THE CHARACTERIZATION AND SURVEILLANCE OF EMERGING PATHOGENS: A STUDY OF FLAVIVIRUS STRAINS INCLUDING THE ZIKA VIRUS

Subhash C. Basak[1,]*, PhD, Marjan Vracko[2], PhD and Ashesh Nandy[3], PhD

[1]Department of Chemistry and Biochemistry,
University of Minnesota Duluth, MN, US
[2]Kemijski institut/National Institute of Chemistry,
Ljubljana, Slovenia
[3]Centre for Interdisciplinary Research and Education,
Kolkata, India

---

* Corresponding Author E-mail: sbasak@nrri.umn.edu.

ABSTRACT

This chapter uses a set of seven alignment-free methods for the characterization of envelope gene sequences of four Flaviviruses, viz., Dengue virus type 2 (DENV 2), West Nile Virus (WNV), Yellow Fefer Virus (YFV), and Zika virus (ZIKV). The sequences are first converted to mathematical objects like graphs, matrices which are subsequently used for the extraction of quantitative sequence descriptors. Such descriptors are then used to calculate intersequence distances like Euclidean distance (ED) and Mahalanobis distance (MD). The utility of such methods of sequence comparison in the characterization of emerging viral pathogens is discussed.

Keywords: Zika virus (ZIKV), Dengue virus type 2 (DENV 2), West Nile virus (WNV), Yellow fever virus (YFV), Microcephaly, IgM antibodies, Basic Local Alignment Search Tool (BLAST) method, Property-activity relationship (PAR), Structure property similaritry principle, Mathematical sequence descriptors, Flavirus envelope genes, Euclidian distance (ED), Mahalanobis distances (MD), Eigenvalues, Analogs, Planar graph, Mapping, Composition, Descriptor function, World Health Organization (WHO), Principal component analysis (PCA)

1. INTRODUCTION

"How is it that you keep mutating and can still be the same virus?"

Chuck Palahniuk, Invisible Monsters

The function of mutation is to maintain the stock of genetic variance at a high level.

Sir Ronald Aylmer Fisher

A recent World Health Organization (WHO) report on priority diseases of public health concern list the following [1]:

- Crimean-Congo hemorrhagic fever (CCHF)

- Ebola virus disease and Marburg virus disease
- Lassa fever
- Middle East respiratory syndrome coronavirus (MERS-CoV) and Severe Acute Respiratory Syndrome (SARS)
- Nipah and Henipaviral diseases
- Rift Valley fever (RVF)
- Zika

The WHO document [1] states: "These diseases pose major public health risks and further research and development is needed, including surveillance and diagnostics".

A combination of their potential to precipitate public health emergencies and the unavailability of effective drugs and/or vaccines necessitates an urgency for accelerated research and development for such diseases.

Zika virus (ZIKV) is one of the priority diseases in the WHO list. ZIKV was first isolated from a febrile rhesus monkey in the Zika forest of Uganda in 1947. For a review, please see chapter 1 of this book. Serosurvey of humans detected ZIKV throughout Africa, Asia, and Oceania. After much global spread of the virus, on 1 February 2016, WHO declared that the association of Zika infection with clusters of microcephaly and other neurological disorders constitutes a Public Health Emergency of International Concern. In November of the same year, however, WHO relaxed this warning.

Confirmation of ZIKV cases are based on (i) detection of ZIKV nucleic acid, detection of ZIKV antigen or isolation of ZIKV from clinical specimens, (ii) detection of ZIKV-specific IgM antibodies in a serum sample and confirmation by neutralization test or (iii) seroconversion or fourfold increase in the titre of ZIKV-specific antibodies in paired serum samples [2, 3].

Comparison of viral nucleic acid sequences provides confirmation of ZIKV infection [4]. The Basic Local Alignment Search Tool (BLAST) method is often used for the comparison of ZIKV sequences with one another. Sequences of NS_5 gene have been used as indicators of the relationship between ZIKV strains [5].

More recently, alignment-free methods have been developed for the representation and characterization of DNA/ RNA/ protein sequences [6-9]. Both planar and non-planar graphs have been used for the representation of sequences. As is well known in the mathematical literature, a graph G is planar if and only if it does not contain a subgraph that is homeomorphic to either K_5 or $K_{3,3}$ [10, 11]. For most molecules [12, 13] and biomolecules like DNA/ RNA sequences and proteins [6-8], the simple planar graph or weighted graph models can be used for the representation of their structure.

2. METHODS

> "It is structure that we look for whenever we try to understand anything. All science is built upon this search; we investigate how the cell is built of reticular material, cytoplasm, chromosomes; how crystals aggregate; how atoms are fastened together; how electrons constitute a chemical bond between atoms. We like to understand, and to explain, observed facts in terms of structure. A chemist who understands why a diamond has certain properties, or why nylon or hemoglobin have other properties, because of the different ways their atoms are arranged, may ask questions that a geologist would not think of' formulating, unless he had been similarly trained in this way of thinking about the world".
>
> *Linus Pauling*

2.1. Characterization of Zika Virus Sequences Using Alignment-Free Descriptors

Alignment-free mathematical descriptors may be used in the characterization of structure (sequence) of viral genomes, either the entire Zika sequence or sequences of NS_5, NS_3, and E genes. Such an approach consists of the following steps:

a) Representation of the viral or gene sequences by corresponding graphs or matrices [6-9],
b) Extraction of quantitative descriptors, e.g., gR or leading eigenvalue of the D/ D matrix as the quantifier of the sequences,
c) Use of the individual sequence descriptor or a set of them to compare sequences with one another or predict their biological properties.

In this chapter we will discuss how sequence descriptors can be used for the comparison of Zika/ Flavivirus gene sequences following the *Structure-Property Similarity Principle.*

2.2. Structure Property Similarity Principle and Sequence Descriptors

"All cases are unique and very similar to the others"

T. S. Eliot, In: The Cocktail Party

"From the words of the poet, men take what meanings please them; yet their last meaning points to thee".

Rabindranath Tagore, Poem #75, Gitanjali

Use of sequence descriptors *vis-à-vis* experimental properties in the comparison of biological properties of sequences like the Zika virus and other Flavivirus genomes or specific gene sequences like those of NS_5, NS_3 or E genes may be clearly understood through a formal exposition of the *structure (sequence) -property similarity principle* [14]. Figure 1 represents an empirical/ experimental property of a sequence as a function $\alpha: C \rightarrow R$ which maps the set C of sequences into the real line R. A non-empirical, sequence based characterization may be looked upon as a composition of a description function $\beta 1: C \rightarrow D$ mapping each sequence in C into a space of non-empirical/ mathematical sequence descriptors (D) and a prediction function $\beta 2: D \rightarrow R$ which maps the descriptors into the real line.

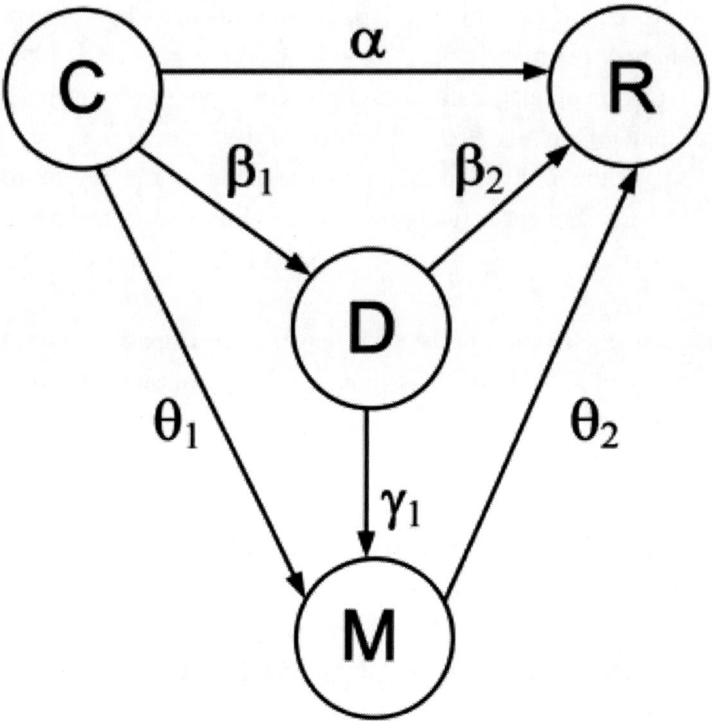

Figure 1. Composition functions for structure-activity relationship (SAR) and property-activity relationship (PAR).

When $[\alpha(C) - \beta 2\ \beta 1(C)]$ is within the range of experimental errors, we say that we have a good predictive model. On the other hand, the property-activity relationship (PAR) is the composition of $\theta 1{:}C \rightarrow M$ which maps the set C into some experimental property space M and $\theta 2{:}M \rightarrow R$ mapping those properties into the real line R. PAR seeks to predict one property (usually a complex property) of a sequence in terms of another (usually simpler) property or a set of properties.

2.3. Sequence Descriptors of Zika and Other Flavivirus Genes

In this section we show an example of how alignment-free mathematical sequence descriptors can be used in the comparison of viral sequences. Table

1 gives the information on four Flavivirus sequences, viz., Dengue virus type 2, West Nile virus, Yellow fever virus, and Zika virus. The data on seven types of computed sequence descriptors, viz., by methods of Nandy, Randic 3D, Wang-Zhang, Ji-Li, Yau, Randic 2D, and Song-Tang, taken from the published paper of Nandy et al. [15] are given in Table 2. One approach of similarity assessment is to compute pairwise distances of objects in n-dimensional spaces, each dimension being represented by one descriptor. Here we have represented the four viral sequences in the 7-dimensional space consisting of the seven computed sequence descriptors and calculated the distances among sequences by two different methods, viz. Euclidean distance and Mahalanobis distance [16]. The mathematical steps, which also include the transformation to principal components, are shown in Tables 3-8.

2.4. Distance Analysis for Four Viruses Described with Seven Descriptors

We calculated the Euclidian and the Mahalanobis distances to origin and distances between objects.

The Euclidian distance (ED) and Mahalanobis distances (MD) are calculated according to equations 1 and 2, respectively.

$$ED^{AB} = \sqrt{\sum_{i=1}^{7}\left(X_i^A - X_i^B\right)^2} \qquad \text{(Eq. 1)}$$

$$MD^{AB} = \sqrt{\left(X_i^A - X_i^B\right)V_{i,j}^{-1}\left(X_j^A - X_j^B\right)} \qquad \text{(Eq. 2)}$$

A, B indicate objects while i, j the running indices over descriptors. V^{-1} is the inverse of covariance matrix.

Data on the viruses and the calculated descriptors used for our analyses are presented in Tables 1 and 2. Four objects are represented with seven descriptors.

Table 1. Information on viral envelope genes

Sequences			Accession no.	Length
Envelope gene (*Flavivirus*)	Dengue virus type 2	DENV2	JX669476	1485
	West Nile virus	WNV	KC601756	1503
	Yellow fever virus	YFV	JN620362	1479
	Zika virus	ZIKV	KX197192	1512

Table 2. Seven sequence descriptors of envelope gene of flaviviruses

Method	Sequence Descriptors				Statistics		
	DENV2	WNV	YFV	ZIKV	Average	SD	SD%
Nandy	72.61	8.91	10.92	4.51	24.24	32.36	133.51
Randic 3D	221.99	113.57	144.37	144.93	156.22	46.24	29.60
Wang-Zhang	43.06	40.08	39.01	24.89	36.76	8.10	22.02
Ji-Li	30.05	42.51	37.93	31.94	35.61	5.69	15.99
Yau	508.81	515.83	507.03	521.15	513.21	6.52	1.27
Randic 2D	1487.07	1505.02	1480.92	1514.01	1496.75	15.39	1.03
Song-Tang	1485.51	1503.43	1479.42	1512.47	1495.21	15.37	1.03

Table 3. Ordered Eigenvalues

Eigenvalue	% of the total variance
3266.676270	86.004%
414.454651	10.911%
117.186432	3.085%
0.000045	negligible
0.000022	negligible
0.000003	negligible
-0.000009	negligible

Table 4. Coordinates of the four viral sequences in the PC space

	PC1	PC2	PC3
DENV2	83.198082	3.057953	3.565636
WNV	-45.427898	-1.529287	13.746897
YFV	-11.774456	-25.568474	-8.593522
ZIKV	-25.995792	24.040104	-8.718920

Table 5. The Euclidean distances between viruses

Virus	Distance to the mean value
DENV2	83.330589
WNV	47.486923
YFV	29.431906
ZIKV	36.465374

Table 6. The pairwise Euclidian distances (distance matrix) between viruses

	DENV2	WNV	YFV	ZIKV
DENV2	0.000000	129.109818	99.935478	111.868065
WNV	129.109818	0.000000	47.005650	39.193283
YFV	99.935478	47.005650	0.000000	51.606907
ZIKV	111.868065	39.193283	51.606907	0.000000

Table 7. The Mahalanobis distances of viruses

Virus	Distance to the mean value
DENV2	2.276778
WNV	2.257351
YFV	2.248449
ZIKV	2.250737

Table 8. The pairwise Mahalanobis distances (distance matrix) between viruses

	DENV2	WNV	YFV	ZIKV
DENV2	0.000000	6.063756	6.032180	6.044493
WNV	6.063756	0.000000	6.001063	5.997902
YFV	6.032180	6.001063	0.000000	5.993867
ZIKV	6.044493	5.997902	5.993867	0.000000

With this data we calculated the Euclidian distances to zero point (average was taken for zero) and distances between objects (viruses), which are shown in distance matrix. The Euclidean distances and the distance matrix are given in Tables 4 and 5. The corresponding Mahalanobis distances and the Mahalanobis distance matrix are in Tables 6 and 7.

3. Results

In the first step we calculated the covariance matrix V and its inverse V^{-1}. It turned out that V is close to singularity which implies that the inverse matrix has extremely high values ($V\ ij \approx 10^7$ and higher). To reduce the intercorrelation within the data we transformed the data into a new system obtained after principal component analysis (PCA). It turned out that the data are almost completely (> 99.99%) described by the first three axes. The percentages of the total variances are shown in Table 3.The new coordinates are shown in Table 4.

Discussion and Conclusions

"As soon as you go into any biological process in any real detail, you discover it's open-ended in terms of what needs to be found out about it".

Joshua Lederberg

"Expect surprises!" should be the watchword of all scientists who try to look beyond the fashions of the day".

Lancelot Law Whyte

In Internal Factors in Evolution (1965),

"Good tests kill flawed theories; we remain alive to guess again".

Karl Popper

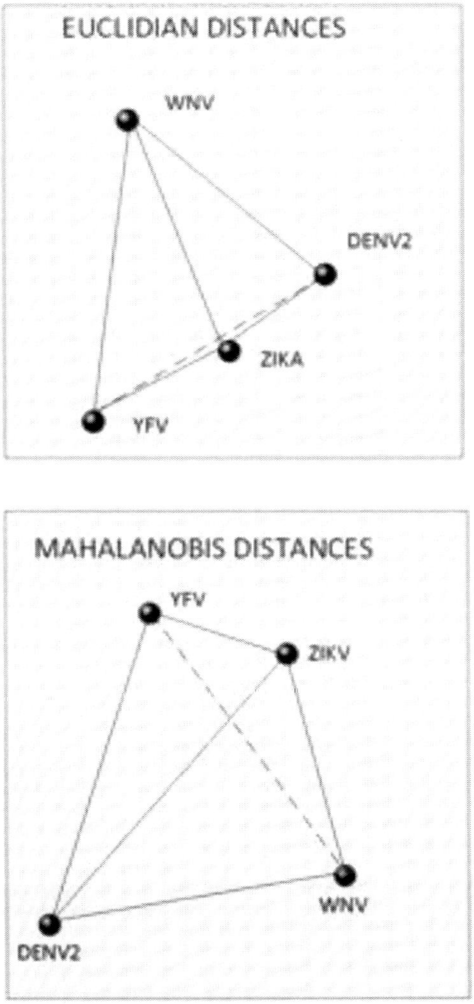

Figure 2A. Representation of pairwise Euclidean and Mahalanobis distances among four viruses represented by sequence descriptors.

The main objective of research results reported in this chapter has been computation of intersequence similarity/ dissimilarity of Flavivirus envelope sequences based on two distance metrics, viz. Euclidena distance and Mahalanobis distance, derived from their seven mathematical sequence descriptors calculated by alignment-free sequence descriptors.

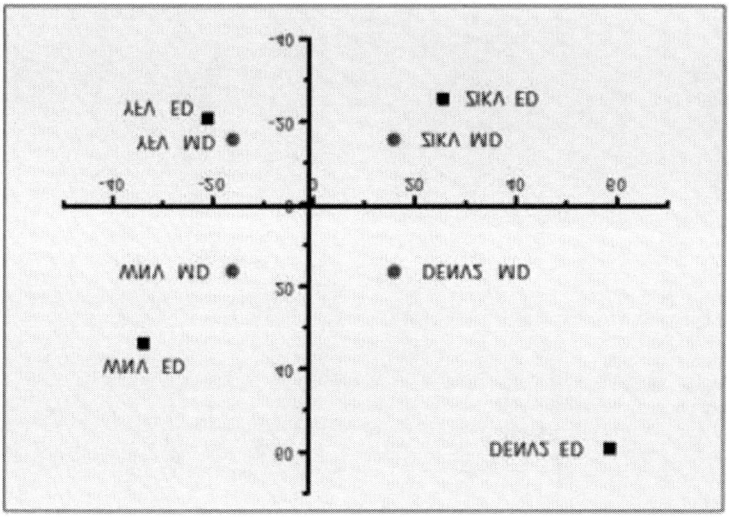

Figure 2B. Shows the distances to the origin. Mahalanobis distances are rescaled by factor 10 (Arbitrary units on x and y axis).

The data in Table 6 shows that in terms of the calculated Euclidean distance DENV is most similar to YFV (ED = 99.93) while it is more dissimilar to WNV (ED = 129.10). In terms of Mahalanobis distance (Table 8), all three viruses, viz., WNV, YFV, and ZIKV seem to be equidistant from DENV (MD = ~ 6 units).

The Euclidian distances show 'eventual similarities' between viruses. However, the Mahalanobis distances show that all objects are equally distant to each other. This means that there is no outliers in the set. In Figure 2A and 2B the four objects are on the edges of tetrahedron.

It has to be emphasized here that the values of the distances vary from one method to another as is evident from the magnitudes of the ED and MD for the four viral sequences. We have tried here to show the potential use of such descriptor based methods taking four viral sequences. As more data become available, such ED and MD methods as well as other distance functions can be applied to sequences to classify them and predict their biological properties.

There is no definite rule for that. Basak et al. [18] developed the idea of 'tailored' similarity space which is geared toward a specific property of interest.

As more experimental properties, both physical and biochemical, become available for sequences, comparative studies of property based vis-a-vis calculated descriptor based similarity methods can be developed. Some research in this area has been done in the past by Basak et al. [19-22].

Finally, we would like to point out that the mathematical descriptor based ED and MD approaches shown in this paper for four viruses may be looked upon as a generic approach of comparing similarity/dissimilarity of sequences from their alignment-free descriptors. Further research is needed to evaluate the usefulness and limitation of this class of methods in the characterization of emerging pathogens and their surveillance.

ACKNOWLEDGMENTS

The authors are thankful to Gregory D. Grunwald, Natrural Resources Research Institute, University of Minnesota Duluth, USA, for collaboration with Subhash C. Basak in various research projects on similarity method development.

REFERENCES

[1] *World Health Organization (WHO) List of Blueprint priority diseases*, http://www.who.int/blueprint/priority-diseases/en/, Accessed on 11 October 2018.

[2] Spiteri, G., Sudre, B., Septfons, A. and Beauté, J. (2017). On behalf of the European Zika surveillance Network. Surveillance of Zika virus infection in the EU/EEA, June 2015 to January 2017. *Euro Surveill,* 22(41):17 - 00254. Accessed October 16, 2018. doi.org/ 10.2807/1560-7917.ES.2017.22.41.17-00254.

[3] Singh, R. K., Dhama, K., Karthik, K., Tiwari, R., Khandia, R., Munjal, A., Iqbal, H. M. N., Malik, Y. S. and Bueno-Marí, R. (2018). Advances in Diagnosis, Surveillance, and Monitoring of Zika Virus: An Update. *Front. Microbiol.*, 8:2677. Accessed October 16, 2018. doi: 10.3389/fmicb.2017.02677.

[4] Zanluca, C., de Melo, V. C., Mosimann, A. L., Dos Santos, G. I., Dos Santos, C. N. and Luz, K. (2015). First report of autochthonous transmission of Zika virus in Brazil. *Mem. Inst. Oswaldo Cruz,* 110:569 – 572. Accessed October 16, 2018. doi: 10.1590/0074-02760150192.

[5] Tognarelli, J., Ulloa, S., Villagra, E., Lagos, J., Aguayo, C., Fasce, R., et al. (2015). A report on the outbreak of Zika virus on Easter Island, South Pacific, 2014. *Arch. Virol.,* 161:665 – 668. Accessed October 16, 2018. doi: 10.1007/s00705-015-2695-5.

[6] Nandy, A. (1994). A new graphical representation and analysis of DNA sequence structure: I. Methodology and Application to Globin Genes. *Current Sci.,* 66:309 - 314.

[7] Nandy, A., Harle, M. and Basak, S. C. (2006). Mathematical descriptors of DNA sequences: development and Applications. *ARKIVOC,* (ix): 211 - 238.

[8] Randić, M., Zupan, J., Balaban, A. T., Vikić-Topić, D. and Plavšić, D. (2011). Graphical representation of proteins. *Chem. Rev.,* 111: 790 - 862.

[9] Seffens, W. (2002). Graph Theory Patterns in the Genetic Codes. *Forma,* 17:309 - 320.

[10] Kuratowski, K. (1930). Sur le probleme des courbes gauches en topologie". *Fundamenta Mathematicae*, 15:271 - 283.

[11] Harary, F. (1969). *Graph theory.* Reading, MA, Addison-Wesley.

[12] Basak, S. C., Magnuson, V. R., Niemi, G. J. and Regal, R. R. (1988). Determining structural similarity of chemicals using graph theoretic indices. *Discrete Appl. Math.,* 19:17 - 44.

[13] Trinajstic N. (1992). *Chemical Graph Theory*, Boca Raton, FL, CRC Press.

[14] Johnson, M., Basak, S. C. and Maggiora, G. (1988). A characterization of molecular similarity methods for property prediction. *Mathl. Comput. Modelling*, 11:630 - 634.

[15] Sen, D., Roy, P., Nandy, A., Basak, S. C. and Das, S. (2018). Graphical representation methods: How well do they discriminate between homologous gene sequences? *Chem. Phys.,* 513:156 - 164.

[16] Mahalanobis, P. C. (1936). On the generalized distance in statistics. *Proceedings of the National Institute of Sciences of India,* 2:49 - 55.

[17] Basak, S. C. and Grunwald, G. D. (1995). Tolerance space and molecular similarity. *SAR QSAR Environ. Res.,* 3:265 - 277.

[18] Basak, S. C., Gute, B. D., Mills, D. and Hawkins, D. M. (2003). Quantitative molecular similarity methods in the property/toxicity estimation of chemicals: A comparison of arbitrary versus tailored similarity spaces. *J. Mol. Struct.: THEOCHEM,* 622: 127 - 145.

[19] Gute, B. D., Grunwald, G. D., Mills, D. and Basak, S. C. (2001). Molecular similarity based estimation of properties: A comparison of structure spaces and property spaces. *SAR QSAR Environ. Res.,* 11:363 - 382.

[20] Gute, B. D. and Basak, S. C. (2001). Molecular similarity-based estimation of properties: A comparison of three structure spaces. *J. Mol. Graphics and Modelling,* 20:95 - 109.

[21] Basak, S. C., Gute, B. D. and Mills, D. (2002). Quantitative molecular similarity analysis (QMSA) methods for property estimation: A comparison of property-based, arbitrary, and tailored similarity spaces. *SAR QSAR Environ. Res.,* 13:727 - 742.

[22] Basak, S. C. (2014). Molecular Similarity and Hazard Assessment of Chemicals: A Comparative Study of Arbitrary and Tailored Similarity Spaces. *J. Eng. Sci. Manage. Educ.,* 7:178 - 184.

Biographical Sketch

Marjan Vračko

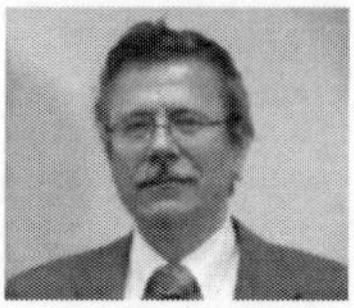

Dr. Marjan Vračko is senior researcher at Kemijski Inštitut/National Institute of Chemistry in Ljubljana, Slovenia. Since 1994 his research is focused to QSAR (quantitative structure-activity relationship) modelling of biological/toxical properties of compounds, to chemometrics (numerical analysis of proteomic and genomic data) and to modeling of interaction between biological receptors and molecules. He is author of over 80 scientific papers, reviews and book chapters.

Publications from the Last 3 Years:

Basak, Subhash C., Vračko, Marjan, Witzmann, Frank A. 2016. "Mathematical nanotoxicoproteomics equantitative characterization of effects of multi-walled carbon nanotubes (MWCNT) and TiO2 nanobelts (TiO2−NB) on protein expression patterns in human intestinal cells." *Current Computer-Aided Drug Design* 12:259-264.

Drgan, Viktor, Župerl, Špela, Vračko, Marjan, Cappelli, Claudia Ileana, Novič, Marjana. 2017. "CPANNatNIC software for counter-propagation neural network to assist in read-across." *Journal of Cheminformatics* 9:1-15.

Drgan, Viktor, Župerl, Špela, Vračko, Marjan, Como, Francesca, Novič, Marjana. 2016. "Robust modelling of acute toxicity towards fathead minnow (Pimephales promelas) using counter-propagation artificial neural networks and genetic algorithm." *SAR & QSAR in Environmental Research* 27:501-519.

Majkovič, Darja, O'Kiely, Padraig, Kramberger, Branko, Vračko, Marjan, Turk, Jernej, Pažek, Karmen, Rozman, Črtomir. 2016. "Comparison of using regression modeling and an artificial neural network for herbage dry matter yield forecasting." *Journal of Chemometrics* 30:203-209.

Plošnik, Alja, Vračko, Marjan, Sollner Dolenc, Marija. 2016. "Mutagenic and carcinogenic structural alerts and their mechanisms of action." *Arhiv za higijenu rada i toksikologiju* 67:169-182.

Ruiz, Patricia, Sack, Alexandra, Wampole, M., Bobst, Sol, Vračko, Marjan. 2017. "Integration of in silico methods and computational systems biology to explore endocrine-disrupting chemical binding with nuclear hormone receptors." *Chemosphere* 178:99-109.

Vračko, Marjan, Basak, Subhash C., Witzmann, Frank A. 2018. "Chemometrical analysis of proteomics data obtained from three cell types treated with multi-walled carbon nanotubes and TiO2 nanobelts". *SAR & QSAR in Environmental Research* 29:567-577.

Vračko, Marjan, Drgan, Viktor. 2017. "Grouping of CoMPARA data with respect to compounds from the carcinogenic potency database." *SAR & QSAR in Environmental Research* 28:801-813.

Chapter 5

DATA-DRIVEN STRATEGIES TO MODEL AND MITIGATE THE THREAT OF ZIKA

Subhabrata Majumdar*

University of Florida Informatics Institute, Gainesville, FL, US

ABSTRACT

The recent outbreak of Zika in Brazil and other Latin American countries has posed several challenges in the domain of public health. Although the outbreak is currently under control, because of the lack of vaccines and drugs till now Zika remains a threat. To effectively formulate strategies for preventing a future outbreak, it is imperative to collate and mine relevant data from different sources. In this direction, several data-driven approaches have been explored. This includes modelling the spread of the disease from past outbreaks, identifying vulnerable geographical areas based on the distribution of mosquito vectors, exploring the virus genome for better understanding of the disease mechanism, screening of chemical compounds as potential targets for drug and vaccine development, and predicting new animal reservoirs of the virus for proactive intervention in the virus life cycle. This chapter explores such strategies in detail: highlighting the major themes of contemporary

---

* Currently at AT&T Labs Research. Corresponding Author E-mail: subho@research.att.com.

research, providing technical discussions and outlining potential directions of future work.

Keywords: Zika, Infectious diseases, SIR (Susceptible-Infectious-Recovered) model, Zika drugs, machine learning, statistical model, Quantitative Structure Activity Relationship (QSAR), disease surveillance

INTRODUCTION

The recent outbreak of the Zika virus (ZIKV) in Brazil and other Latin American countries has posed several challenges in the domain of public health. Even though the epidemic that originated in 2015-16 is mostly over, and projected incidence rates are low even in all large cities in Latin American Countries (LAC) (O'Reilly et al. 2018), this threw up a lot of challenges and inadequacies. After the first confirmed case was reported in Brazil in 2015, the number of suspected cases in Brazil only was put at 440,000-1,300,000 that year (Zanluca et al. 2015). It still remains a mystery that how a relatively unknown flavivirus managed to spread across a vast geographic region in such a small amount of time. This suggests our limited knowledge about the obscure infectious diseases, and underscores the need for detailed investigation into the different aspects of diseases like, but not limited to, Zika: the disease spread mechanism, early detection and forecasting of infection spread, and detection of new vectors and reservoirs of the virus.

For the above purposes, quantitiative modelling approaches have been explored for a number of diseases, e.g., the severe acute respiratory syndrome (SARS) (Dye and Gay 2003), middle-east respiratory syndrome (MERS) (Chowell et al., 2014), Dengue (Andraud, et al. 2012, Bakach and Braselton 2015) and Ebola (Chretien, Riley and George 2015). Fortunately, a considerable part of the flurry of research activities during and after the ZIKV outbreak has been devoted to mathematical and data-driven models of phenomenon that encompass known approaches like incidence modelling and forecasting (Wiratsudakul, Suparit and Modchang 2018), as well some new avenues, like predicting new vectors or animal reservoirs (Evans et al. 2017, Han et al. 2018), and exploration of the ZIKV genome (Dey et al. 2017).

Overview of Approaches

This chapter outlines and elaborates on the major lines of quantitative approaches focused on countering ZIKV. We devote the second section to mathematical modelling of disease spread. Here we start from the well-known Susceptible-Infectious-Recovered, or SIR, model and expand its modifications and expansions to effectively model the spread of ZIKV. The following section is devoted to data-driven models. Due to the availability of high computational power and internet, there is more scope to access and leverage different data sources, like genomic, clinical and epidemiological data. Linking these disparate sources and gathering insights from them within the first few days of an outbreak is key to effective disease surveillance (Holmes, Rambaut and Andersen 2018). Motivated by this, we elaborate on different aspects of quantitative methods that can supplement conventional clinical surveillance: exploration of the viral genome, detecting new disease carrier animals, screening of potential chemical compounds for drug development using computational models, and using secondary information sources, like social media, internet search trends, for early detection of an outbreak. Following this, in the next section we give a list of the major freely available Zika-related data sources for interested researchers, and give possible future directions of research. Finally, we conclude the chapter by summarizing our discussion and underlining the relevance of quantitative approaches.

MATHEMATICAL MODELS

The Basic SIR Model

The (Susceptible-Infectious-Recovered) SIR model is perhaps the most widely used mathematical models for modelling the spread of infectious diseases (Hethcote 2000, Keeling and Danon 2009, Vynnycky and White 2010). Here each individual in a population is considered to fall in one of the three categories-

a) *Susceptible (S):* healthy individuals who are susceptible to infections.
b) *Infectious (I):* Diseased individuals who are capable of transmitting the pathogen to someone in the S group,
c) *Recovered (R):* Individuals with past infections that have recovered and are immune to future infections.

At time point *t*, the SIR model is defined by the following differential equations that give rates of changes between these categories:

$$\frac{dS}{dt} = -\frac{\beta IS}{N},$$
$$\frac{dI}{dt} = \frac{\beta IS}{N} - \gamma I,$$
$$\frac{dR}{dt} = \gamma I,$$

where β is the transmission rate of the disease from an infectious to susceptible individual, and γ is the recovery rate of an infected person. This model has seen widespread and successful application in modelling the spread of several infectious diseases, and several variations to account for situations like mortality, population growth, vector-borne transmission etc. Detailed literature reviews of research on SIR models, their extensions and relevance in real-life disease modelling can be found in Hethcote 2000, Vynnycky and White 2010, Huppert and Katriel 2013, and Bauer 2017.

An important component of SIR models is the *basic reproduction number*, which is generally denoted by the notation R_0. This is defined as the average number of infections an infected person causes among the susceptible population during the time they are infected. A high R_0 means the disease is likely to spread, whereas a small value indicates the infection is likely to subside after a certain time. In our basic SIR model above, R_0 is denote by the ratio of infection rates, i.e., β/γ (Rock et al. 2014). With this definition, $R_0 > 1$ would mean the spread of the infection, and vice versa. However the SIR model needs to be modified to better model different infectious diseases, and the expression of R_0 would depend on the specific model formulation.

SIR Modelling for Zika

There are two main modes of transmission of the Zika virus: a) through mosquitos, i.e., vector-borne, and b) sexual (the minor modes include laboratory contamination (Centers for Disease Control and Prevention 2017) and blood transfusion (Musso et al. 2014)). In the first case, the *Aedes aegypti* and *Aedes albopictus* mosquitos are vectors of the virus: which have markedly different behavioral pattern, biting preferences and chance of harboring ZIKV (Garcia-Luna et al. 2018). Since both mosquitos feed on humans mostly during daytime, they have a high chance of exposure to humans. Consequently, biting rate can have a seasonal component depending on weather and climate patterns. (Suparit, Wiratsudakul and Modchang 2018) Modified the traditional SIR model to incorporate this scenario. They start with formulating two parallel SIR models for the human and mosquito populations, and assume rates of transmission between the S, I and R classes of these populations that account for seasonal variations. From their analysis of ZIKV infection data in Bahia, Brazil, Suparit, Wiratsudakul and Modchang 2018 observed a strong positive correlation between temperature and their estimated biting rates, validating previous related studies on other infectious diseases. Under this model, the values for several geographical regions were calculated by H. Nishiura et al. 2016a, 2016b and Shutt et al. 2017.

ZIKV can also be transmitted sexually, and leads to microcephaly in the children of infected pregnant women (Mlakar et al. 2016, Agusto, Bewick and Fagan 2017, Padmanabhan, Seshaiyer and Castillo-Chavez 2017) extended the SIR model to account for this mode of transmission. Both of the studies extend the basic model to account for other types of individual. Padmanabhan, Seshaiyer and Castillo-Chavez 2017 worked within the framework of the SEIR model (Hethcote 2000), which introduces an extra Exposed (E) category, containing susceptible individuals that are actually exposed to infected persons. They considered an SEIR model for humans, SEI model for mosquito vectors, and construct their differential equations taking into account both sexual and vector transmissions. Within this framework, they estimated the basic reproduction number R_0, and consider the effects of remediation efforts like mosquito nets and spraying. Agusto, Bewick and Fagan 2017 further extended the SEIR model to focus on mother-to-child transmission. They broke down the human population into babies and adults, considered different rates for each sub-population, and incorporated the categories asymptomatic, Symptomatic newborn but without and with microcephaly within the babies and asymptomatic and symptomatic categories within the adults. They also consider a range of remediation efforts within this model, and conclude that using protection during sex while being infected with ZIKV is more effective in preventing microcephaly than focusing on mosquito reduction. However, controlling both avenues of infection have positive effects in restricting the spread of the disease (Srivastav, et al. 2018).

Among other explorations in ZIKV involving the SIR model, Goswami et al. 2018 moved away from the linear formulation of differential equations in the SIR model and its variants to propose a human-vector SIR model with non-linear incidence rates. Finally, Wang et al. 2017 considered remediation of Zika by introducing *Wolbachia* bacteria into the mosquitos and built this into their set of SIR-type differential equations, and Caminade et al. 2017 revealed the possible influence of the 2015-16 El-Niño climate phenomenon behind the outbreak. A comprehensive list of other similar approaches for modelling ZIKV spread can be found in Table 1 of Wiratsudakul, Suparit and Modchang 2018.

Non-Compartmental Models

All the approaches underlined in the previous section operate at the population level, or as called in the infectious disease literature, are compartmental models (May and Anderson 1991, Capasso 1993). However, infectious disease spread is significantly affected by a number of factors, such as spatio-temporal effects, network effects and even variations at the individual level. This calls for the use of more involved models that can vary for disease to disease.

For ZIKV, the factors affecting disease incidence, like mosquito biting rate, temperature, and human density vary considerably across geographical locations and seasons. In addition, climate change has significantly altered the dynamics of how infectious diseases spread (Agan 2017). Thus the integration of spatio-temporal effects in ZIKV models to gain the correct insights about disease spread and forecasting future spreads is essential. To this end, a spatial differential equation-based model was proposed by Fitzgibbon, Morgan and Webb 2017. In one of the largest data-analytic exercises involving ZIKV, Perkins et al. 2016 predicted the epidemic spread trajectory at a local level among childbearing women in the South American continent. They estimated several parameters, e.g., mosquito mortality, human-to-mosquito transmission rate, from a modified SIR model, and plugged them into a deterministic model to calculate the ratio for ZIKV infection in mothers at locations across continental South America. To this end, they used highly granular population data (Sorichetta et al. 2015), and data on historical temperature patterns (Hijmans et al. 2005). In an unpublished manuscript, Perkins et al. 2018 explored spatial differences of disease spread trajectories across several locations in Colombia.

For network-based models, movement patterns of individuals, airline route maps and movement of livestocks serve as reliable proxies for contact within individuals or groups of individuals (Wiratsudakul, Suparit and Modchang 2018). Based on this concept, Saad-Roy, Van den Driessche and Ma 2016, and Scata et al. 2016 explored the effect of human connection networks on ZIKV and microcephaly incidence.

The final factors affecting transmission patterns of ZIKV are variations that are specific to individuals or groups of them, and are not accounted for by spatio-temporal or network factors. Metapopulation models work within the framework of the SIR model defined above, considering parallel models for different sub-populations. The works of Baca-Carrasco and Velasco-Hernandez 2016, and Zhang et al. 2017 are important in this context. The individual-level agent-based models are generally more computationally intensive. Using agent-based frameworks, Matheson, Satterthwaite and Highlander 2017 modeled the spread of ZIKV during the 2016 Olympics among different population groups such as tourists and locals, and Kuhlman et al. 2018 modeled the ZIKV outbreak in Miami, USA in 2016.

Data-Driven Modelling

At present, the ZIKV infection is at an endemic stage, thus it is an ideal time to study its characteristics from several angles (Goswami et al. 2018). Besides proposing modelling disease spread and validating them using past infection data, there is scope to better understand the behavior of the disease and the virus itself using quantitative approaches in other areas as well. This includes better forecast of disease spread using social media data, predicting new wild reservoirs of ZIKV, using *in silico* computer models to identify candidates for vaccine development (See chapter 3 for the development of a set of candidates for peptide vaccine). With the large amount of public health data available on the internet and the advancement of high-performance computing, the time is ripe to mine and analyze data related to each of the above diverse goals, and work towards a coherent understanding of ZIKV infection.

In this section, we discuss recent research efforts in this direction. We divide the possible insights gleaned from quantitative approaches into three categories: Inference about the disease mechanisms, progress on development of vaccines, and forecasting future outbreaks.

Data-Driven Inferences

Understanding the transmission mechanism and the structure of ZIKV, as well as devising strategies for vector management are essential for keeping the ZIKV in control (Arora, Banerjee and Narasu 2018). There are several sources of data that can be utilized for this purpose. The genetic and behavioral data can be used for gaining insight towards the vectors, genetic data related to different virus strains can be used to characterize ZIKV better, and structural descriptors pertaining to chemical compounds can be used to train algorithms that detect potential candidates for vaccine development.

The transmission of ZIKV is a two-stage process. ZIKV resides in the wild within certain primate species, who themselves do not get infected, and transmit the virus from generation to generation. In the first stage, the virus gets transmitted from these reservoir animals to mosquito vectors when they bite the animals. In the second stage, humans get infected by the mosquito vectors that carry the virus from these reservoirs or other humans (Figure 1). There are only two confirmed reservoirs of ZIKV, and two mosquito vectors that are able to acquire and transmit the virus (WHO Regional Office for Europe 2016). However, the virus has been isolated from several other species, and its similar transmission pattern compared to other flaviviruses (e.g., Dengue, West Nile Virus) brings the vectors of these diseases into scrutiny as well. Motivated by this, Evans et al. 2017 used publicly available data on mosquito and virus characteristics and machine learning methods to predict potential new vectors of ZIKV. According to their finding, more than two-third of potential ZIKV vectors are yet to be identified, and 25+ additional species are likely contributors in ZIKV transmission. On the other hand, Han et al. 2018 used Bayesian statistical methods and known reservoir status of primates that are known reservoirs for other flaviviruses to identify potential new reservoirs. A number of species that they detected as potential reservoirs, e.g., the white-fronted capuchin (*Cebus albifrons*) and

Venezuelan red howler (*Alouatta seniculus*) monkeys live in close proximity to humans or are even kept as pets. Such situations provide potential explanations for the sudden explosion of ZIKV outbreak in Brazil and surrounding countries, and call for more focus and investigation.

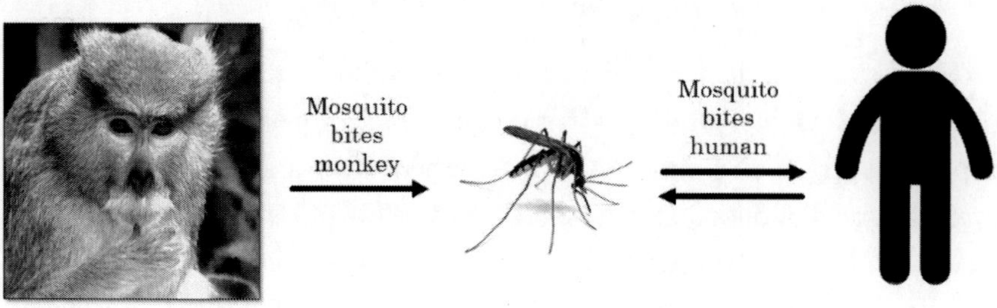

Figure 1. Transmission path of ZIKV: virus gets transmitted from wild reservoir primates to mosquitoes, then humans. Mosquitos can also bite infected humans and transmit the virus to other humans.

Drug Development

The biochemistry of different strains of the virus provides another piece in decoding the puzzle of ZIKV transmission. To this end, Nandy et al. 2016 gave a complete characterization of the Zika viral genome by analyzing gene sequence data of all available ZIKV strains. According to their findings, the Zika virus is genetically close to the Dengue virus, and the strain responsible for the latest outbreak in South America is structurally different from the older Africa strain. Following this, Dey et al. 2017 identified a number of common segments across the sequencing data of these strains and obtained four peptide segments through a screening procedure that can potentially help design ZIKV vaccines. On a similar note, Ekins et al. 2016a developed homology-based models for all 15 proteins on the surface of ZIKV and identify potential structures in these compounds that can be exploited for drug or vaccine development.

Because of the limited knowledge on the mechanistic and structural properties of ZIKV, effective drugs or vaccines remain elusive, and prevention of the disease is solely based on remediation. Since the number of potential candidates for any drug is huge, computational models to perform *in silico* screening in order to narrow down the candidate for further scrutiny are needed. This Quantitiative Structure Activity Relationship (QSAR) approach has been a major part of the last few decades. After the ZIKV outbreak in Brazil, a few studies have taken this route to discover new vaccine candidates for the virus. For drugs to be used in clinical treatment, multiple studies have identified a number of compounds that act as inhibitors of RNA polymerase (Singh and Jana 2017, Pattanaik et al. 2018, Elfiky and Ismail 2018), NS3 protease (Bhargava et al. 2017, Sahoo, et al. 2016, Yuan et al. 2017) and NS5 protease (Ramharack and Soliman 2018) enzymes present in ZIKV. Interestingly, due to similarities of how ZIKV works inside the body with other diseases, there is potential for existing drugs to be repurposed for developing drugs against Zika (Devillers 2018, Mesci et al. 2018, Balasubramanian et al. 2017). A detailed discussion of ZIKV-related *in silico* approaches can be found in Sinigaglia, et al. 2018.

Forecasting the Spread of ZIKV

Even though the current Zika outbreak is mostly over (O'Reilly et al. 2018), it remains a global public health threat, and sporadic cases keep coming up: for example the very recent incidences reported in Rajasthan, India (NDTV 2018). The studies of Evans et al. 2017, and Han et al. 2018 point to the fact that there are potentially more unknown vectors and reservoir primates that are vehicles of ZIKV transmission. Because of these reasons, considerable focus must be put on forecasting future incidences of Zika infection.

During the ZIKV outbreak in Brazil, Zinszer et al. 2017 predicted the spatial trajectory and speed of spread of the virus through Brazil, while Bogoch et al. 2016a built a forecasting model for its spread internationally that integrates different factors such as seasonal variation and travel patterns. In one of the largest ZIKV studies until now in terms of spatial scale, Messina et al. 2016 predicted environmental suitability of ZIKV infection in different parts of the world. They used ZIKV occurrence data with latitude and longitude information and environmental covariates, e.g., precipitation, humidity, forest cover, and used boosted regression tree-based predictive model to obtain probability heatmaps for large areas in the Americas (central and south), Africa (central and west) and Asia (south and south-east). According to their findings, all of these regions contain high-probability areas that are conducive to future ZIKV incidences. However, based on *Aedes* mosquito population projections, it is unlikely to spread to Europe (Guzzetta et al. 2016).

In addition to environmental variables, there are other data sources that can be utilized. Bogoch et al. 2016b explored the potential of ZIKV spread in Africa and Asia-pacific by modelling and identified high-probability regions by analyzing data collected from a number of sources. They accounted for the spread of Zika from South America by considering airline transportation data, and in conjunction with mosquito occurrence and environmental data, obtained predicted probabilities of ZIKV introduction at different months across the year, and a number of locations using boosted regression trees. Lo and Park 2018 showed using tools from topological data analysis that how geographical locations can be weighted using mosquito density and human population data and used in conjunction with environmental variables for ZIKV infection forecasting.

Forecasting models are valuable in predicting early detection of future ZIKV spreads and identifying potential geographical hotspots from where the infection is spreading. Chowell et al. 2016 showed that even simple phenomenological models built on past count data can be effective in early detection. According to the findings of Chien et al. 2018, weather measurements like humidity, temperature and rainfall are predictive of future incidence of Zika cases. Internet and social media are also effective in this respect. Web search queries have been shown to be effective in infectious disease surveillance (Chan et al. 2011, Alicino et al. 2015). According to the findings of Brown et al. 2018, during the 2016 ZIKV outbreak in Colombia high volumes of google search trends for the word 'Zika' systematically preceded number of reported cases. The crucial takeaway from such studies is that there is scope of using unconventional data sources like internet search trends, weather variables to supplement and strengthen conventional clinical surveillance of ZIKV incidences.

Discussion

Data Sources

From the host of modelling activities described above and the insights gained from them, it is clear that data-driven quantitative approaches are essential in combating the Zika menace. To achieve this goal, diverse datasets describing different facets of the behavior of ZIKV, e.g., disease incidence, mosquito abundance, weather, demographic data, genomic information etc. need to be easily available and accessible to researchers. However this is not always the case- in general for infectious diseases (Chretien, Rivers and Johansson 2016), and *especially* for Zika (Siraj et al. 2018) because of its relatively unknown status until the last few years. Furthermore, many of the studies we mention integrate different data sources in order to build a richer model (Bogoch et al. 2016b, Messina et al. 2016, Han et al. 2018). The availability of central repositories for data sources are absolutely essential to undertake such efforts. In the early days of ZIKV infection, this availability of such data were scarce. But fortunately, due to efforts from multiple concerned agencies like the World Health Organization (WHO) and the United States Centers for Disease Control and Prevention (CDC), several data repositories are freely available on the internet now. We summarize them in Table 1.

A few other specific data sources are given in Table 1 of Ekins et al. 2016b. Furthermore, curated datasets merging multiple data sources are available through individual papers, like Siraj et al. 2018.

Table 1. The main public data sources for Zika

Name	Link	Short description
CDC Zika Data Repository	https://github.com/cdcepi/zika	Central repository about publicly available datasets all over the internet. Divided country-wise.
BuzzFeed Zika Data Guide	https://github.com/BuzzFeedNews/zika-data	Contains data and pointers to Zika related data: divided country-wise as well as
Zika Open-Research Portal	https://www.re3data.org/repository/r3d100012059	A common collaboration space and data portal for Zika researchers

Future Directions

The flurry of research activities following the 2015-16 outbreak of Zika is an encouraging sign. There is ample evidence that data driven modelling can translate to more effective management of the spread of the disease, as seen during the 2014-15 Ebola outbreak (Meltzer et al. 2014, Bellan et al. 2015), and a few instances for Zika as well (Zhang et al. 2017). There are two aspects of future research: expanding on our current knowledge and understanding of ZIKV, and using similar approaches to predict other emerging infectious diseases.

The predictive models we discussed indicate that the potential for Zika outbreaks further in future remain because of a large number of potentially unknown vectors and reservoirs (Evans et al. 2017, Han et al. 2018). More such studies need to be performed for a better grasp of the scenario, as there is dearth of literature in the case of Zika because of its relative unknown status till now (Vorou 2016). Even though data sources are available, collecting and joining different sources of data is often a nontrivial task due to internal inconsistencies and missing data (Siraj et al. 2018, Han et al. 2018). A more involved approach focused on data mining, missing data imputation etc. that leverage expertise of researchers from quantitative fields is needed to tackle this fundamental problem.

Secondly, there is scope of reusing the mathematical models and algorithms to predict incidences of other diseases. In the early days of the 2015-16 outbreak, Rodriguez-Barraquer et al. 2016 showed that incidences of other arboviruses can be used to predict intensities of ZIKV infection. A number of comparative analysis of ZIKV and dengue have pointed out their similarities (Nandy et al. 2016, Funk et al. 2016, Suwanmanee and Luplertlop 2017). Since dengue is much more widespread and is a continuing menace (Bhattacharya et al. 2013, Ganeshkumar et al. 2018), ZIKV modelling efforts can strengthen and inform the fight against dengue with additional insights.

CONCLUSION

Prediction of infectious diseases is a multi-pronged approach. Even though many computational avenues are available to shed more light on diseases, there is an ongoing conversation about the veracity, or even need for them: especially in spending public health budget to fund research on data analytic solutions instead of surveillance (Holmes, Rambaut and Andersen 2018, Yong 2017). To underline the importance of data and modelling approaches in this conversation, there is a need for properly communicating the results of such studies to policymakers. The sudden outbreak of ZIKV tells us about the myriad of factors affecting the disease spread we know little or nothing about, and the research efforts we mention in this chapter give some sense of direction in this situation. Thus Zika provides an ideal scenario in the larger public health dialog where data-driven prediction and clinical surveillance can work together and strengthen each other in combating future threats.

An interdisciplinary approach, drawing on the expertise of domain experts in areas such as disease ecology, public health, statistics/machine learning, is needed for quantitative models to be effective. To this end, a higher participation of methodology researchers is required. Out-of-the-box machine learning tools are often not effective in modelling the specific problems in real-world disease datasets, such as missing data (Han et al.

2018) and positively unlabeled problems (Jowkar and Mansoori 2016), and higher involvement of methodology experts will help navigate these problems to gather effective and actionable insights from the data that are more likely to convince policymakers about the efficacy of these methods.

ACKNOWLEDGMENT

The author was supported by Prof. George Michailidis during his time in University of Florida Informatics Institute.

REFERENCES

Agan, P. N. 2017. "Climate Change and Health Nexus: A Review." *J. earth Sci. Clim. change* 8 (12): 1000435.

Agusto, F. B., S. Bewick, and W. F. Fagan. 2017. "Mathematical model of Zika virus with vertical transmission." *Infect. Dis. Model.* 23 (2): 244-267.

Alicino et al., C. 2015. "Assessing Ebola-related web search behaviour: insights and implications from an analytical study of Google Trends-based query volumes." *Infect. Dis. Poverty* 4: 54.

Andraud, M., N. Hens, C. Marais, and P. Beutels. 2012. "Dynamic Epidemiological Models for Dengue Transmission: A Systematic Review of Structural Approaches." *PLoS One* 7 (11): e49085.

Arora, N., A. K. Banerjee, and M. L. Narasu. 2018. "Zika outbreak aftermath: status, progress, concerns and new insights." *Future Virol.* 13 (8): 539-556.

Baca-Carrasco, D., and J. X. Velasco-Hernandez. 2016. "Sex, mosquitoes and epidemics: an evaluation of Zika disease dynamics." *Bull. Math. Biol.* 78: 2228-2242.

Bakach, I, and J. Braselton. 2015. "A Survey of Mathematical Models of Dengue Fever." *J. Comput. Sci. Syst. Biol.* 8: 255-267.

Balasubramanian et al., A. 2017. "Antiviral activities of selected antimalarials against dengue virus type 2 and Zika virus." *Antiviral Res.* (137) 141-150.

Bauer, F. 2017. "Mathematical epidemiology: Past, present, and future." *Infect. Dis. Model.* 2 (2): 113-127.

Bellan et al., S. E. 2015. "Statistical power and validity of Ebola vaccine trials in Sierra Leone: a simulation study of trial design and analysis." *Lancet Infect. Dis.* 15 (6): 703-710.

Bhargava et al., S. 2017. "Identification of structural requirements and prediction of inhibitory activity of natural flavonoids against Zika virus through molecular docking and Monte Carlo based QSAR Simulation." *Nat. Prod. Res.* in press. doi: https://doi.org/10.1080/14786419.2017.1413574.

Bhattacharya et al., M. K. 2013. "Dengue: A Growing Menace -- A Snapshot of Recent Facts, Figures & Remedies." *Int. J. Biomed. Sci.* 9 (2): 61-67.

Bogoch et al., I. I. 2016a. "Anticipating the international spread of Zika virus from Brazil." *Lancet* 387 (10016): 335-336.

Bogoch et al., I. I. 2016b. "Potential for Zika virus introduction and transmission in resource-limited countries in Africa and the Asia-Pacific region: a modelling study." *Lancet Infect. Dis.* 16 (11): 1237-1245.

Brown et al., M. 2018. "Modeling Zika Virus Spread in Colombia Using Google Search Queries and Logistic Power Models." *bioRxiv.* doi: https://doi.org/10.1101/365155.

Caminade et al., C. 2017. "Global risk model for vector-borne transmission of Zika virus reveals the role of El Niño 2015." *Proc. Natl. Acad. Sci. USA* 114 (1): 119-124.

Capasso, V. 1993. *Mathematical Structures of Epidemic Systems.* Berlin: Springer-Verlag.

Centers for Disease Control and Prevention 2017. *Laboratory Safety when Working with Zika Virus.* 4 27. https://www.cdc.gov/zika/laboratories/lab-safety.html.

Chan et al., E. H. 2011. "Using Web Search Query Data to Monitor Dengue Epidemics: A New Model for Neglected Tropical Disease Surveillance." *PLoS Negl. Trop. Dis.* 5 (5): e1206.

Chien et al., L.-C. 2018. "Surveillance on the endemic of Zika virus infection by meteorological factors in Colombia: a population-based spatial and temporal study." *BMC Infect. Dis.* 18 (1): 180.

Chowell et al., G. 2014. "Synthesizing data and models for the spread of MERS-CoV, 2013: Key role of index cases and hospital transmission." *Epidemics* 9: 40-51.

Chowell et al., G. 2016. "Using Phenomenological Models to Characterize Transmissibility and Forecast Patterns and Final Burden of Zika Epidemics." *PLoS Curr.* 8.

Chretien, J.-P., C. M. Rivers, and M. A. Johansson. 2016. "Make data sharing routine to prepare for public health emergencies." *PLoS Med.* 13: e1002109.

Chretien, J.-P., S. Riley, and D. B. George. 2015. "Mathematical modeling of the West Africa Ebola epidemic." *eLife* 4: e09186.

Devillers, J. 2018. "Repurposing drugs for use against Zika virus infection." *SAR QSAR Environ. Res.* 29: 103-115.

Dey et al., S. 2017. "A Bioinformatics approach to designing a Zika virus vaccine." *Comput. Biol. Chem.* 68: 143-152.

Dye, C., and N. Gay. 2003. "Modeling the SARS Epidemic." *Science* 300 (5627): 1884-1885.

Ekins et al., S. 2016a. "Illustrating and homology modeling the proteins of the Zika virus." *F1000Res.* 5: 275.

Ekins et al., S. 2016b. "Open drug discovery for the Zika virus." *F1000Res.* 5: 150.

Elfiky, A. A., and A. M. Ismail. 2018. "Molecular docking revealed the binding of nucleotide/side inhibitors to Zika viral polymerase solved structures." *SAR QSAR Environ Res.* 29 (5): 409-418.

Evans et al., M. V. 2017. "Data-driven identification of potential Zika virus vectors." *eLife* 6: e22053.

Fitzgibbon, W.E., J.J. Morgan, and G.F. Webb. 2017. "An outbreak vector-host epidemic model with spatial structure: the 2015-2016 Zika outbreak in Rio De Janeiro." *Theor. Bio. Med. Model.* 14 (7): 1-17.

Funk et al., S. 2016. "Comparative Analysis of Dengue and Zika Outbreaks Reveals Differences by Setting and Virus." *PLoS Negl. Trop. Dis.* 10 (12): e0005173.

Ganeshkumar et al., P. 2018. "Dengue infection in India: A systematic review and meta-analysis." *PLoS Negl. Trop. Dis.* 12 (7): e0006618.

Garcia-Luna et al., S. M. 2018. "Variation in competence for ZIKV transmission by Aedes aegypti and Aedes albopictus in Mexico." *PLoS Negl. Trop. Dis.* 12 (7): e0006599.

Goswami et al., N. K. 2018. "Mathematical modeling of zika virus disease with nonlinear incidence and optimal control." *J. Phys. Conf. Ser.* (IOP Publishing) 1000: 012114.

Guzzetta et al., G. 2016. "Assessing the potential risk of Zika virus epidemics in temperate areas with established Aedes albopictus populations." *Euro. Surveill.* 21 (15): 30199.

Han et al., B. 2018. "Confronting data sparsity to identify potential sources of Zika virus spillover infection among primates." *Epidemics*, in press.

Hethcote, H. 2000. "The Mathematics of Infectious Diseases." *SIAM Review* 42 (4): 599-653.

Hijmans et al., R. 2005. "Very high resolution interpolated climate surfaces for global land areas." *Int. J. Climatol.* 25: 1965-1978.

Holmes, E. C., A. Rambaut, and K. G. Andersen. 2018. "Pandemics: spend on surveillance, not prediction." *Nature* 558: 180-182.

Huppert, A., and G. Katriel. 2013. "Mathematical modelling and prediction in infectious disease epidemiology." *Clin. Microbiol. Infect.* 19 (11): 999-1005.

Jowkar, G. H., and E. G. Mansoori. 2016. "Perceptron ensemble of graph-based positive-unlabeled learning for disease gene identification." *Comput. Biol. Chem.* 64: 263-270.

Keeling, M. J.; and L. Danon. 2009. "Mathematical modelling of infectious diseases." *Br. Med. Bull.* 92: 33-42.

Kuhlman et al., C. J. 2018. "Hybrid Agent-based modeling of Zika in the united states." *2017 Winter Simulation Conference (WSC).*

Lo, D., and B. Park. 2018. "Modeling the spread of the Zika virus using topological data analysis." *PLoS ONE* 13 (2): e0192120.

Matheson, T., B. Satterthwaite, and H. C. Highlander. 2017. "Modeling the spread of the Zika virus at the 2016 olympics." *Spora: A Journal of Biomathematics* 3: 29-44.

May, R. M., and R. M. Anderson. 1991. *Infectious diseases of humans: dynamics and control.* Oxford: Oxford University Press.

Meltzer et al., M. E. 2014. "Estimating the future number of cases in the Ebola epidemic--Liberia and Sierra Leone." *MMWR Suppl.* 63: 1-14.

Mesci et al., P. 2018. "Modeling neuro-immune interactions during Zika virus infection." *Hum. Mol. Genet.* 27 (1): 41-52.

Messina et al., J. P. 2016. "Mapping global environmental suitability for Zika virus." *eLife* 5 (1): e15272.

Mlakar et al., J. 2016. "Zika virus associated with microcephaly." *New Eng. J. Med.* 374: 951-958.

Musso et al., D. 2014. "Potential for Zika virus transmission through blood transfusion demonstrated during an outbreak in French Polynesia, November 2013 to February 2014." *Euro. Surveill.* 10 (19): 14.

Nandy et al., A. 2016. "Characterizing the Zika Virus Genome – A Bioinformatics Study." *Curr. Comput. Aided Drug. Des.* 12: 87-97.

NDTV. 2018. *3 Fresh Zika Cases In Rajasthan Takes Total To 126.* October 22. https://www.ndtv.com/india-news/3-fresh-zika-cases-in-rajasthan-takes-total-to-126-1935892.

Nishiura et al., H. 2016a. "Transmission potential of Zika virus infection in the South Pacific." *Int. J. Infect. Dis.* 45: 95-97.

Nishiura et al., H. 2016b. "Preliminary estimation of the basic reproduction number of Zika virus infection during Colombia epidemic, 2015–2016." *Trav. Med. Infect. Dis.* 14: 274-276.

O'Reilly et al., K. M. 2018. "Projecting the end of the Zika virus epidemic in Latin America: a modelling analysis." *BMC Medicine* 16: 180.

Padmanabhan, P., P. Seshaiyer, and C. Castillo-Chavez. 2017. "Mathematical modeling, analysis and simulation of the spread of Zika with influence of sexual transmission and preventive measures." *Lett. Bioinform.* 4 (1): 148-166.

Pattanaik et al., A. 2018. "Discovery of a non-nucleoside RNA polymerase inhibitor for blocking Zika virus replication through in silico screening." *Antiviral Res.* 151: 78-86.

Perkins et al., T. A. 2016. "Model-based projections of Zika virus infections in childbearing women in the Americas." *Nat. Microbiol.* 1 (9): 16126.

Perkins et al., T. A. 2018. "What lies beneath: a spatial mosaic of Zika virus transmission in the 2015-2016 epidemic in Colombia." *bioRxiv* 276006. https://www.biorxiv.org/content/early/2018/03/05/276006.

Ramharack, P., and M. E. S. Soliman. 2018. "Zika virus NS5 protein potential inhibitors: an enhanced in silico approach in drug discovery." *J Biomol. Struct. Dyn.* 36 (5): 1118-1133.

Rock et al., K. 2014. "Dynamics of infectious diseases." *Rep. Prog. Phys.* 77: 26602.

Rodriguez-Barraquer et al., I. 2016. "Predicting intensities of Zika infection and microcephaly using transmission intensities of other arboviruses." *Bull. World Health Organ.* doi:10.2471/BLT.16.174128.

Saad-Roy, C. M., P. Van den Driessche, and J. Ma. 2016. "Estimation of Zika virus prevalence by appearance of microcephaly." *BMC Infect. Dis.* 16: 754.

Sahoo, M., L. Jena, S. Daf, and S. Kumar. 2016. "Virtual Screening for Potential Inhibitors of NS3 Protein of Zika Virus." *Genomics Inform.* 14 (3): 104-111.

Scata et al., M. 2016. "The impact of heterogeneity and awareness in modeling epidemic spreading on multiplex networks." *Sci. Reports* 6: 37105.

Shutt et al., D. P. 2017. "Estimating the reproductive number, total outbreak size, and reporting rates for Zika epidemics in South and Central America." *Epidemics* 21: 63-79.

Singh, A., and N. K. Jana. 2017. "Discovery of potential Zika virus RNA polymerase inhibitors by docking-based virtual screening." *Comp. Biol. Chem.* 71 (C): 144-151.

Sinigaglia, A., S. Riccetti, M. Trevisan, and L. Barzon. 2018. "In silico approaches to Zika virus drug discovery." *Expert Opin. Drug Discov.* 13 (9): 825-835.

Siraj et al., A. S. 2018. “Spatiotemporal incidence of Zika and associated environmental drivers for the 2015-2016 epidemic in Colombia.” *Sci. Data* 5: 180073.

Sorichetta et al., A. 2015. “High-resolution gridded population datasets for Latin America and the Caribbean in 2010, 2015, and 2020.” *Sci. Data* 2: 150045.

Srivastav, A. K., N. K. Goswami, M. Ghosh, and X.-Z. Li. 2018. “Modeling and optimal control analysis of Zika virus with media impact.” *Int. J. Dynam. Control* in press. doi: https://doi.org/10.1007/s40435-018-0416-0.

Suparit, P., A. Wiratsudakul, and C. Modchang. 2018. “A mathematical model for Zika virus transmission dynamics with a time-dependent mosquito biting rate.” *Theor. Biol. Med. Model.* 15: 11.

Suwanmanee, S., and N. Luplertlop. 2017. “Dengue and Zika viruses: lessons learned from the similarities between these Aedes mosquito-vectored arboviruses.” *J. Microbiol.* 55 (2): 81-89.

Vorou, R. 2016. “Zika virus, vectors, reservoirs, amplifying hosts, and their potential to spread worldwide: what we know and what we should investigate urgently.” *Int. J. Infect. Dis.* 48: 85-90.

Vynnycky, E., and R.G. White. 2010. *An Introduction to Infectious Disease Modelling.* Oxford: Oxford University Press.

Wang, L., H. Zhao, S. M. Oliva, and H. Zhu. 2017. “Modeling the transmission and control of Zika in Brazil.” *Sci. Rep.* 7: 7721.

WHO Regional Office for Europe 2016. *Zika virus vectors and risk of spread in the WHO European Region.* http://www.euro.who.int/data/assets/pdf_file/0007/304459/WEB-news_competence-of-Aedes-aegypti-and-albopictus-vector-species.pdf?ua=1.

Wiratsudakul, A., P. Suparit, and C. Modchang. 2018. “Dynamics of Zika virus outbreaks: an overview of mathematical modeling approaches.” *PeerJ* 6: e4526.

Yong, E. 2017. *Is It Possible to Predict the Next Pandemic?* Oct 25. https://www.theatlantic.com/science/archive/2017/10/pandemic-prediction-challenge/543954/.

Yuan et al., S. 2017. "Structure-based discovery of clinically approved drugs as Zika virus NS2B-NS3 protease inhibitors that potently inhibit Zika virus infection in vitro and in vivo." *Antiviral Res.* 145: 33-43.

Zanluca et al., C. 2015. "First report of autochthonous transmission of Zika virus in Brazil." *Mem. Inst. Oswaldo Cruz* 110: 569-572.

Zhang et al., Q. 2017. "Spread of Zika virus in the Americas." *Proc. Natl. Acad. Sci. USA* 114: 433-443.

Zinszer et al., K. 2017. "Reconstruction of Zika Virus Introduction in Brazil." *Emerg. Infect. Dis.* 23 (1): 91-94.

BIOGRAPHICAL SKETCH

Subhabrata Majumdar

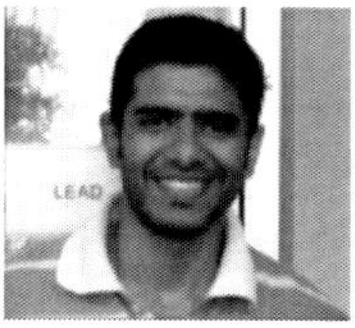

Subhabrata Majumdar is a postdoctoral researcher in the University of Florida Informatics Institute, where he works on developing data integration methods for of complex omics data using high-dimensional graphical models. His ongoing projects include exploring statistical foundations of artificial intelligence and uncertainty quantification in complex high-dimensional systems. He has a PhD in statistics from the University of Minnesota Twin Cities, where his dissertation covered development of statistical methods based on data depth, focusing on dimension reduction and variable selection. Subhabrata has extensive experience in applied statistical research, with past and present collaborations spanning diverse areas like climate science, statistical chemistry, behavioral genetics and public health, and has an ongoing interest in the social and ethical aspects of data science and machine learning.

Publications from the Last 3 Years:

Basak, S. C., and S. Majumdar, S. 2016. "Editorial: Chemodescriptor Based QSARs of Structurally Homogeneous Versus Heterogeneous Chemical Data Sets: Some Comments on the Congenericity Principle vis-à-vis Diversity Begets Diversity Principle." *Curr. Comput. Aided Drug Des.* 12: 84-86.

Biswas, T., and S. Majumdar. "Statistical Methods: Need for a Rethink." *Indian Pediatrics* 54: 65.

Majumdar, S., and S. C. Basak. 2016. "Exploring intrinsic dimensionality of chemical spaces for robust QSAR model development: A comparison of several statistical approaches." *Curr. Comput. Aided Drug Des.* 12: 294-301.

Majumdar, S., and S. C. Basak. 2018. "Beware of external validation! – A Comparative Study of Several Validation Techniques used in QSAR Modelling". *Curr. Comput. Aided Drug Des.* 14: 284-291.

Majumdar, S., and S. C. Basak. 2018. "Editorial: Beware of Naïve q^2, use True q^2: Some Comments on QSAR Model Building and Cross Validation." *Curr. Comput. Aided Drug Des.* 14: 5-6.

Majumdar, S., and S. Chatterjee. "Nonconvex penalized multitask regression using data depth-based penalties." *Stat* 7: e174.

Majumdar, S., S. C. Basak, C. N. Lungu, M. V. Diudea, and G. D. Grunwald. 2018. "Mathematical structural descriptors and mutagenicity assessment: A study with congeneric and diverse data sets." *SAR QSAR Environ. Res.* 29: 579-590.

ABOUT THE EDITORS

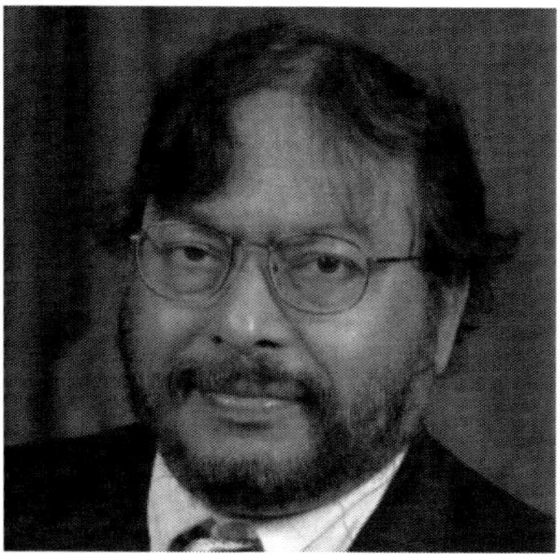

Subhash C. Basak received his PhD in biochemistry in 1981 from the University of Calcutta, India. He was a faculty research Associate in the Department of Chemistry, University of Minnesota-Duluth, during 1982-1987. Subsequently, during 1987-1911 Basak was a Senior Scientist at the Natural Resources Research Institute (NRRI) and Adjunct Professor in the Department of Chemistry, Biochemistry, and Molecular Biology. He is currently Adjunct Professor in the Department of Chemistry and Biochemistry, University of Minnesota-Duluth. Basak's research areas during the past four decades have been: 1) Biochemistry of psychoactive drugs, 2) Drug tolerance, 3) Structure-activity relationship of drugs and toxicants using mathematical structural descriptors, 4) Development of

Novel Topological Indices, 5) Hierarchical QSAR (quantitative structure-activity relationship), 6) Quantitative Molecular Similarity Analysis (QMSA) Methods, 7) Development of novel DNA/ RNA Sequence descriptors and applications, 8) Mathematical Proteomics, 9) Characterization of molecular chirality using Relative Chirality Index (RCI), 10) Modelling in Nanotoxicoproteomics, 11) Characterization of drug addiction, 12) Differential quantitative structure-activity relationship (DiffQSAR) for drug resistance, 13) Statistical methods in QSAR, and 14) Philosophy of mathematical chemistry. He is currently the Editor-in-Chief of the international journal Current Computer Aided Drug Design. He is also past President of the International Society of Mathematical Chemistry.

For details of Basak's publications, please see:

https://www.researchgate.net/profile/Subhash_Basak

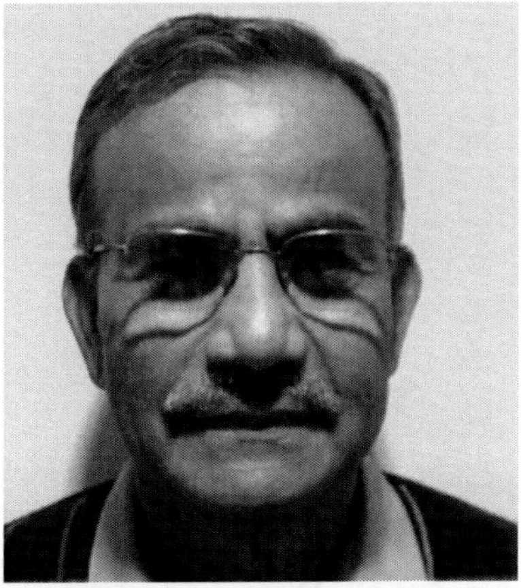

Dr. Apurba K Bhattacharjee is currently an Adjunct Professor at the Department of Microbiology and Immunology at the School of Medicine, Georgetown University, Washington, DC, U.S.A. Earlier he was a Senior Scientist (Chief Molecular Modeler) at the Walter Reed Army Institute of Research, Maryland, (U.S.A.) from where he retired in 2015. He held a Ph.D. from NEHU, India and a postdoc for three years from the Institute of Topology and Dynamics of Systems (Paris, France) under Professor J.-E. Dubois. Dr. Bhattacharjee has over 30 years of research experience in

Computer Assisted Drug Design (CADD), particularly in the application of quantum chemistry, pharmacophore modeling, and virtual screening of compound databases in the discovery of bioactive agents. His background of physical chemistry and quantum chemistry in particular enables him to a deep understanding of different algorithms for specific computations. His focus on Molecular Electrostatic Potentials (MEPs) of bioactive compounds and application of the idea in pharmacophore modeling led him to many successful design and discovery of potential therapeutic agents. His current research interest is in the field of antivirals targeting specifically the dengue and Zika viruses. He has authored and coauthored 130 peer reviewed international publications including several book chapters and five patents.

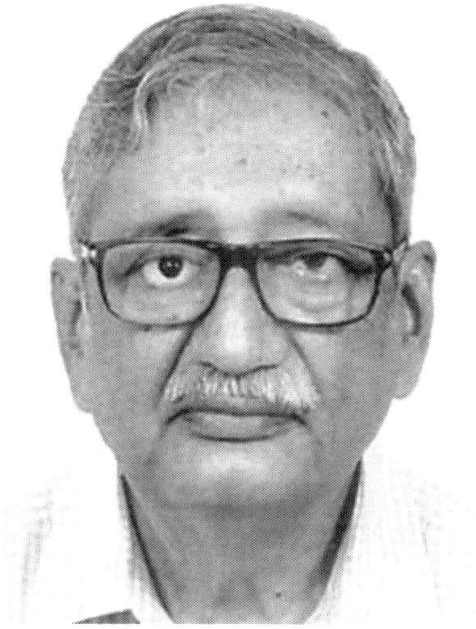

Dr Ashesh Nandy did his PhD in Quantum Electrodynamics in 1971 from the University of California, Santa Barbara, Calif., USA and post-Doc at Syracuse University, Syracuse, New York and Max Planck Institute for Biophysical Chemistry at Göttingen, Germany. Returning to India in 1975, he joined the Indian Association for Cultivation of Science and later the Indian Institute of Chemical Biology. There he developed his model for graphical representation of DNA sequences and pursued the work there and later in Jadavpur University. In 2005-6 he worked on a project at the Natural

Resources Research Institute, Duluth, Minnesota, USA developing his approach to designing vaccines for viral diseases using graphical and mathematical models on viral sequences which continues to this day. He has published numerous papers in national and international peer reviewed journals and written several book chapters.

INDEX

#

A

B

C

D

E

F

G

H

I

J

K

L

M

N

O

P

Q

R

S

Z

Zika Virus Disease: Prevention and Cure

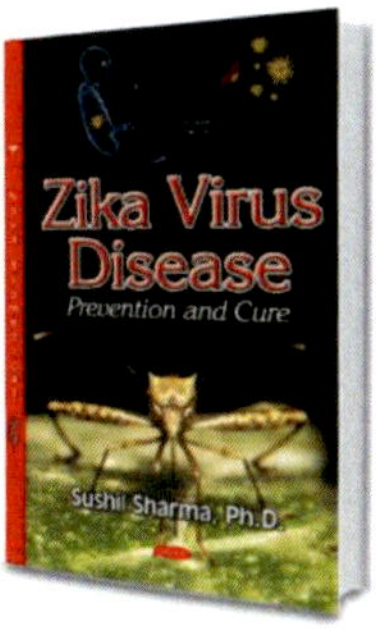

Author: Sushil K. Sharma, Ph.D.

Series: Virology Research Progress

Book Description: The author was motivated to write this important book because currently there is no systematically-written document on the ZIKV disease, which could serve at this crucial moment as a textbook for medical students, physicians, nurses, and other healthcare providers as well as a reference book for basic researchers, professors, and the general public.

Hardcover ISBN: 978-1-53610-769-2
Retail Price: $230

Dengue Virus: Detection, Diagnosis and Control

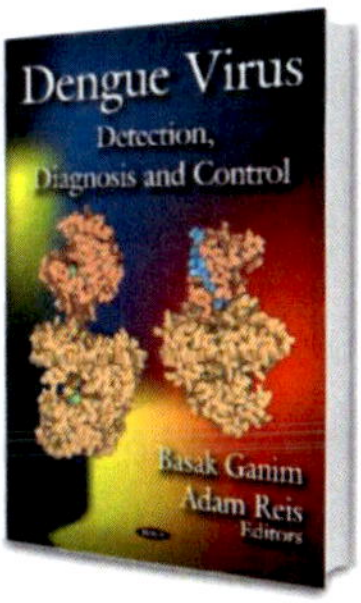

Editors: Basak Ganim and Adam Reis

Series: Virology Research Progress

Book Description: This book aims to review the possible molecular mechanisms that attribute to the variation of Dengue virus (DENV) disease.

Hardcover ISBN: 978-1-60876-398-6
Retail Price: $280

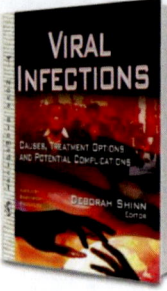